Making Information
Technology Work

Making Information Technology Work

Maximizing the Benefits for Health Care Organizations

Roger Kropf, PhD
Guy Scalzi, MBA

Health Forum, Inc.
An American Hospital Association Company
CHICAGO

AHA
press

Printed in the United States of America—09/07

Cover design by Tim Kaage

ISBN: 978-1-55648-349-3

Item Number: 093001

Discounts on bulk quantities of books published by Health Forum, Inc., are available to professional associations, special marketers, educators, trainers, and others. For details and discount information, contact Health Forum, Inc., One North Franklin, 28th Floor, Chicago, IL 60606-3421 (Phone: 1-800-242-2626).

Library of Congress Cataloging-in-Publication Data

Kropf, Roger.
   Making information technology work : maximizing the benefits for health care organizations / Roger Kropf and Guy Scalzi.
      p. ; cm.
   Includes bibliographical references and index.
   ISBN 978-1-55648-349-3
   1. Health services administration—Information technology.   2. Medical care—Information technology.   3. Health facilities—Information services.   4. Information resources management.   I. Scalzi, Guy. II. Title.
   [DNLM: 1. Medical Informatics.   2. Health Facilities—organization & administration.   3. Information Management—organization & administration.   W 26.5 K93m 2007]
   RA971.23.K76 2007
   362.1068—dc22
                                                         2007023867

To Marcia and Claudia

Contents

List of Figures and Tables

About the Authors

Roger Kropf, PhD, is a professor in the Health Policy and Management Program at New York University's Robert F. Wagner Graduate School of Public Service. Dr. Kropf is the author of two previous books on the application of information systems to health care management. *Strategic Analysis for Hospital Management* was written with James Greenberg, PhD, and published by Aspen Systems in 1984. *Service Excellence in Health Care through the Use of Computers* was published by the American College of Healthcare Executives in 1990. He teaches graduate and executive education courses on information technology. More information on his work can be found at www.wagner.nyu.edu/kropf and his Web site, www.nyu.edu/classes/kropf.

Guy Scalzi, MBA, is executive vice president of Velōz Global Solutions. From 2000 to 2005, he was senior vice president and managing director of First Consulting Group's Management Services business. He has held the position of chief information officer at the New York-Presbyterian Health Care System; New York/Cornell Medical Center; and the Hospital for Joint Diseases, a division of New York University Medical Center. In 1985, he became one of the founders of a software development company, DataEase International. With Guy Scalzi as president, this venture capital–funded start-up grew rapidly and in 1990 was sold to a consortium of its distributors. He moved to Europe to head international operations and continued growing DataEase's presence throughout Europe, Asia, and South America. Guy Scalzi was also a hospital administrator at St. Vincent's Medical Center, Bellevue Hospital, and Montefiore/Einstein Medical Center in New York for fourteen years.

Preface

ALL HEALTH CARE managers are involved in the use of information technology (IT). They may be involved in deciding which projects will be implemented: their budgets are the source of funds, or the IT expenditure replaces spending on projects they value. The days when IT could be considered the exclusive domain of the IT department are over.

Despite their investment in IT projects, managers are often not sure how to manage new or existing projects. Many managers are not knowledgeable about the technical elements of information technology and may even feel reluctant to learn, believing that IT is a complex "black box" best left to those who are technically trained. Managers often are uncomfortable becoming involved in monitoring the level of human and financial resources devoted to a major IT project or its timeline for completion. This reluctance leads to many IT projects being over budget and often far behind schedule. Managers also may never be sure if the benefits that were expected are actually achieved.

This book explores the before, during, and after of IT implementation. How should we decide what to invest in? How can implementation be managed so that the chances of success are increased? How can we find out if we got the benefits that were expected—and increase the chances of success the next time? This book explores tools that managers can use to become involved and to improve the chances of effective implementation of IT that supports organizational objectives and provides value. The tools are used before, during, and after project implementation—a cycle that is repeated many times as changes occur in the organization's IT infrastructure.

The intended audience for this book is health care managers in hospitals, health systems, and large physician practices. This includes chief executive officers, chief operating officers, and department- and service level managers at the corporate and individual hospital levels. The book will also be a valuable resource for students in health administration and management programs.

How This Book Is Organized

In part I, we focus on how benefits are estimated before making an investment in IT. This requires considering the financial impact, process improvements, and intangible benefits of the investment. Intangible benefits are those that cannot easily be expressed in dollar terms, such as improved patient and staff satisfaction. A number of methods for doing a benefits study are explained, and methods for carrying out a financial analysis are described. The steps in creating a business plan to support a recommendation are then defined.

In part II, we define the components of project management, which include scope, time, cost, communications, and integration management. Without tight project management, an organization's projects are in constant jeopardy of missing their targets. The need for a project management office (PMO) is explained, along with the various PMO models that can be implemented. Project and portfolio management software is an important tool, and the types that are available are explained, along with considerations in making a purchase.

Having defined benefits at the beginning, managers need to ensure that benefits are received at the end. In part III, we explore what should happen after an IT implementation. We describe how a post-implementation audit can be carried out by comparing pre- and post-implementation performance, conducting time and motion studies, and studying pilot installations.

Finding Key Points in This Book

This book includes a number of features that will help those try-ing to grasp key points. Throughout the book, readers will find

---

Text in boxes to emphasize important points.

In addition, the introduction to each of the three parts of the book includes recommendations—

What All Hospitals Should Be Doing

—as well as a discussion of important decisions that need to be made.

Roger Kropf
Guy Scalzi

Acknowledgments

W E WANT TO thank the people who took time out of their very busy lives to help us develop case studies for the book.

- Tom Zenty and Ed Marx at University Hospitals in Cleveland
- Judy Van Norman at Banner Health in Phoenix
- George Brenckle at the University of Pennsylvania Health System in Philadelphia
- John Shufeldt and Tracy Patterson at NextCare Urgent Care in Phoenix

Help in writing the cases was also provided by staff of several consulting and vendor organizations. Gregg Mohrmann and Rinette Scarso from First Consulting Group helped us better understand the challenges of project management and project management offices. Bill Weber of First Consulting Group explained how service level agreements work from the vendor's viewpoint. Kevin Ford from Cerner Corporation and Ben Wilson from Intel assisted in the development of the Banner Estrella case study.

Brad Kirkman-Liff from Arizona State University and Brian Malec from California State University at Northridge deserve our thanks for their help in finding organizations willing to work with us in writing case studies.

Steve Finkler from the Wagner School at New York University, Will Ferniany from the University of Mississippi Medical Center, George Vecchione from Lifespan, Bruce Schroffel from the University of Colorado Medical Center, and Alex and Sheila Szafran from Maine Medical Center all provided comments that improved the book.

We also want to thank Neil Jesuele, executive vice president of the American Hospital Association, for his support of the project.

Finally, we want to thank our editor at AHA Press, Richard Hill, for his efficiency and guidance during the entire publication process.

Introduction

Major Tasks for Managers

> **Health care managers need to get involved in IT projects from beginning to end to ensure a successful outcome.**

HEALTH CARE managers have three major tasks that are necessary to obtain value from investments in information technology (IT):

- Benefits definition
- Project management
- Benefits realization

Benefits Definition

Defining and agreeing on what *value* means is essential to success. Resources are scarce, and IT competes with other worthwhile investments. Senior management should be able to report what benefits were received. This is not a trivial task, since IT projects may be undertaken for multiple reasons and some of the benefits are hard to measure. Financial return on investment (ROI) is one type of value, but IT projects may be undertaken not because they deliver a high financial return but to improve clinical quality and patient safety. Even when financial ROI is the primary value sought, estimating the financial return may not be easy. Some returns such as reduced document storage costs are more certain than others, such as reduced labor costs. How is the value of projects that provide the infrastructure required for other projects to be estimated? Health care managers need to lead their organizations to select and use measures of value and implement the systems required to measure value before making an investment.

In part I, we examine how benefits are estimated before making an investment in IT. This requires considering the financial impact, process improvements, and intangible benefits of the investment. Intangible benefits are those that cannot easily be expressed in dollar terms, such as improved patient and staff satisfaction. A number of methods for doing a benefits study are explained, as are methods for carrying out a financial analysis. The steps in creating a business plan to support a recommendation are then described.

Project Management

Information technology is widely considered by health care managers to be difficult to implement. Information technology implementation requires the involvement of senior management and professional project management. This means putting in place a structure for project governance to decide what projects should be undertaken, who is responsible for them, how changes will be made, and what resources will be used. Management means bringing together a team of trained project managers to monitor progress and create systems that collect and make accessible information on progress. It usually requires selecting a software tool that enables the collection, analysis, and communication of information on projects.

In part II, we define the components of project management as it is defined by the Project Management Institute, the principal organization that certifies professionals in the field. These components include scope, time, cost, communications, and integration management. The need for a project management office (PMO) is explained, along with the various PMO models that can be implemented. Project and portfolio management (PPM) is an important tool; the types of PPM are explained, along with considerations in making a purchase.

Benefits Realization

Part III explores what should happen after IT implementation. We describe how a post-implementation audit can be carried out by comparing pre- and post-implementation performance, conducting time and motion studies, and studying pilot installations.

What can we do to get the benefits that were expected? Benefits are not automatically achieved because the project is completed and systems work as planned. Information technology that produces labor savings does not necessarily result in fewer staff and lower labor costs or current staff redirecting their time to another valuable activity. Having defined benefits at the beginning, managers need to ensure that those benefits are achieved. This requires a plan for achieving them and ongoing analysis of what was actually obtained.

Formal benefits realization processes that seek to define and manage the attainment of benefits are described in part III. This often involves the creation of special teams and the definition of who is accountable for achieving each benefit. Some organizations have also developed written contracts called service level agreements (SLAs) with an external vendor or an internal IT department. We define SLAs and how they can be negotiated and used internally. We consider the possible positive and negative effects of SLAs, how they can be measured, and what costs are involved.

A Health Care Manager's Role in Selecting and Implementing Information Technology

Ultimately the benefits of IT will only be achieved if health care managers work with their in-house staff, staff from outsourcing companies (if one of them is being used), and the vendors whose products they purchase. We offer some advice on how to make that relationship more rewarding.

Role Working with In-House Information Technology

Health care managers need to take the steps described below to create effective working relationships with in-house IT staff.

Be involved in every step of the IT selection and implementation process. Health care managers need to examine each iteration of the product as it is tested and customized to meet their needs—or it will not. They need to be willing to change the processes in their units and not become wedded to what was done in the past. The implementation of IT correctly brings with it the desire to improve the efficiency of processes that may have been in place for a long time. Getting the full benefits of IT means changing how work is done.

Accept accountability for achieving the benefits from IT. Technology enables the achievement of benefits, but those benefits result from the work of clinicians and other staff and their willingness to use the technology and to make changes in how they work. If they will not use the technology and will not change, the benefits will not be achieved. Unit or department managers—not IT staff—are accountable for the behavior of their staffs and for producing the changes needed.

Be champions for the technology and the process changes that are implemented. If managers are indifferent, the implementation will fail and the benefits will not be achieved. Clinical and other staff need to know that managers support the implementation of IT and believe the stated benefits can be gained.

Provide the resources they committed to providing. The time of clinical and other staff is needed during the entire selection and implementation process. If that time is promised but not delivered, then the implementation cannot proceed on schedule. For example, if a schedule for training is agreed on, then clinical staff need to be available at the agreed-upon times.

Role Working with Outsourcing Companies and Vendors

The staffs of outsourcing companies and vendors are not the enemy. If managers choose to enter into a contract, they have accepted those companies as part of the team. Creating a "we-them" polarization impedes the work to be done. The resources of both outsourcing companies and vendors should be used. They are the ones who have done the work before, and managers can learn from them. Otherwise, managers are not getting the value their organizations paid for.

Aren't People Important?

Much of this book advocates adopting systems, processes, and procedures. This is not because we believe that focusing on people—involving them and helping them to deal with change—is unimportant; we believe it is critical to success. But much has been written about how to work with physicians, nurses, and other health care professionals when IT projects are undertaken. Less has been said about how such projects should be managed. Information technology projects require *both* the application of change management and human relations skills as well as methodologies for defining value, project management, and getting the value desired. If people are forgotten, we can wind up using project management skills to drive the project to failure as clinicians resist implementation. It may be "on time, on budget," but it will still be a failure.

Information Technology Project Selection

Information technology projects compete with other investments for scarce capital. A typical process for selecting a project is:

- The project sponsor asks the IT department to evaluate vendors/solutions.
- Vendors and/or methodologies for solutions are proposed and evaluated.
- Rough cost estimates are calculated for two or three solutions.
- The list is narrowed down to one, and a final cost estimate is completed.
- Return on investment is calculated, including "hard" tangible savings and "soft" intangible savings.
- A senior organizational committee prioritizes all requests, including those that are IT related.
- The list is matched against available funds, and finalists are selected.

The case that follows illustrates how one health system chose to select and implement IT. It describes the governance process that has been established to allocate limited capital and to make managers—not the IT department—accountable for success and the achievement of the benefits described during the project selection process. University Hospitals in Cleveland, Ohio, has chosen to establish a PMO and hire professional project managers to help ensure that implementation is a success. It has created a "closed loop" process, which requires that project sponsors return after implementation and put the benefits proposed and those achieved side by side, providing a powerful incentive for working to achieve those benefits.

Case Study No. 1

University Hospitals: Information Technology Governance and the Creation of a Project Management Office

Introduction

University Hospitals (UH) is a multi-hospital system with head-quarters in Cleveland, Ohio (www.uhhospitals.org). Senior management has instituted changes in information technology governance and project management that have resulted in an increase in the percentage of IT projects that are on time and on budget from 50 percent to 90 percent in three years. The changes included the creation of a project management office (PMO) operated by First Consulting Group (FCG). First Consulting Group handles day-to-day operation of all of University Hospitals's IT resources.

University Hospitals

University Hospitals includes a 947-bed, tertiary care medical center, Case Medical Center, and seven community hospitals with 891 beds. It has 3 million outpatient visits and 110,000 inpatient discharges annually. It is the primary affiliate of Case Western Reserve University School of Medicine.

University Hospitals consolidated its IT resources in one organization in 2000. The Information Technology and Solutions (IT&S) department is viewed as an "enterprise resource," so one IT staff handles technology needs for the entire system. University Hospitals outsourced day-to-day operations to FCG in 2002. Chief information officer (CIO) Ed Marx and four division information officers (DIOs) maintain UH employee status. First Consulting Group created a PMO, which is currently staffed by eight project managers (PMs) and a PMO director.

Marx believes that UH has dramatically improved its on-time, on-budget rate for IT projects from a 50 percent rate to a 90 percent rate. This has been accomplished by changes in IT governance and how projects are managed, including the creation of the PMO.

Information Technology Governance

Tom Zenty III, UH's chief executive officer (CEO), believes great dissatisfaction exists in hospitals with IT projects because little ownership is taken by the operations user. Those users expect the leader of the IT function to tell them what they need and to make it happen. When Zenty came to UH, there was not a high level of support for IT because people were turning over that responsibility to an IT leader and were not getting the kind of results they were expecting. The IT people felt that operations was disengaged from implementation of IT projects, and the operations people felt that IT was functioning with complete autonomy and independence. Zenty believes this is a "recipe for failure." So Zenty and Marx created an IT steering committee. Zenty said he was going to expect ownership, buy-in, and support from those in operations. Accountability is also required from the IT function, and expectations need to be managed.

Marx defines *IT governance* as "exercising authority or control over the decision to utilize IT resources in pursuit of organizational objectives or strategies," or "how decision rights and accountabilities are distributed and shared between business and IT executives." Governance defines "how IT decisions are made, who gets to make them, who has input, and who is accountable for what."

An IT steering committee and four IT advisory committees were created for the IT governance structure. The advisory committees are for ambulatory, clinical and business systems, and IT infrastructure. Projects that were considered IT projects (because they involved computer hardware and software) are no longer considered to belong to IT&S. They are projects of the operating units that have been identified as subject to the IT governance process. The Information Technology and Solutions department is the enabler but not the owner of projects, with the exception of IT infrastructure projects such as expansion or upgrade of computer storage. Even after becoming operational, the systems still belong to the operating units. The IT&S staff provides technical support such as hardware and computer network maintenance.

The IT steering committee, with Zenty as chair and Marx as co-chair, meets bimonthly. Members include the chief operating officer, chief financial officer (CFO), and senior vice president of strategy at UH in addition to the CEO and CFO of the academic medical center and a practicing physician. The purposes of the steering committee are to ensure that UH is using its limited resources in a way that supports its strategy and to create a single process for reviewing, approving, prioritizing, and funding projects.

The governance process provides a single intake process that makes projects easier for the customer. Before the changes, the different processes and entry points resulted in many service requests and projects that were understaffed, mismanaged, or even lost, causing a rising rate of dissatisfaction with IT&S services within the user community.

Marx believes the new governance process takes away all the ambiguity in how to get a project done. It also helps to ensure IT alignment with core business units. In the past, people could get any project approved through a variety of routes, including legal, supply chain, finance, or IT&S, regardless of whether it was the best investment for UH and was aligned with the vision of the organization. When Marx became CIO, he says, "We had 300 applications, all sorts of hardware platforms. It was just a mess."

Strategic Alignment

Vision 2010 is UH's strategic plan for the next five years. One of the plan's priorities is to create an electronic health record (EHR). A five-year IT plan is also now in place to support Vision 2010. Once a year, the IT steering committee meets to review a list of proposed projects; this process is called the "recalibration of the IT project portfolio," in light of UH's strategic plan. The recalibration session is a four-hour meeting at which IT&S acts as a facilitator. For 2007, $250 million worth of requests were submitted for IT projects. Approximately 20 percent of UH's total capital budget is related to IT and would go through the IT governance process. (This does not include the major $100 million EHR initiative.)

Requests for projects are first approved by a senior vice president, who reviews a "preliminary scope" document that includes the affected entities, funding source, desired completion date, realistic completion date, and cost estimate. The scope document (or a business plan for projects more than $100,000) is completed by the PMO. Projects are presented to one of the advisory committees, which makes a recommendation. Figure CS1-1 shows the elements contained in a scope document.

About 150 projects pass through this process and are reviewed at the annual steering committee "big board" meeting. A card representing each project, which has previously been categorized according to one of the seven corporate strategies and placed in that category (e.g., patient safety) is rank ordered and placed on the board using Velcro. The committee has a total available budget for IT projects and must decide which projects will go forward for the following year and which will be postponed. Each project has an executive sponsor—one of the ten senior vice presidents—who presents to the committee a one-page summary of the capital and operating cost and rationale for the project related to UH's strategy.

Boards are also available for each year beginning with the next for the following six years (e.g., 2007–2012). Projects are discussed, and a decision is reached on which year the project should go forward. A staff member with a spreadsheet keeps track of the impact on the capital budget of adding and removing projects from the board for the following year. Permissible total capital spending is the primary constraint forcing prioritization. When total spending is exceeded, vigorous debate takes place about which projects should be postponed.

Figure CS1-1.   Contents of a Project Scope Document

A.   Current Environment
B.   Project Scope Statement and Activities
C.   Project In-Scope Activities
D.   Project Out-of-Scope Activities
E.   Business Objectives
F.   Assumptions
G.   Training Needs
H.   Ongoing Support
I.   Regulatory Impact
J.   Network Assessment
K.   Budget Breakdown
L.   High-Level Timeline
M.   Deliverables
N.   Dependencies
O.   Risk Points
P.   Roles and Responsibilities
Q.   Strategic Alignment
R.   Dependent Documents
S.   Other Critical Documents Needed
T.   Vendor List
U.   Project Identification Statement
V.   Signatures
W.   Operating-Level Agreement

Source: University Hospitals, Information Technology & Solutions, Case Medical Center Anesthesiology, Scope Document, CL-1065, November 30, 2005. Reprinted with permission from University Hospitals, Cleveland, Ohio.

Project Management Office

University Hospitals's PMO is operated by staff of First Consulting Group, the organization to which UH has outsourced day-to-day IT operations. Once a project is approved by the IT steering committee, it goes to the PMO director who assigns a project manager. The PM then uses the project scope or business plan approved by the steering committee to enter a budget, timeline, and work breakdown structure (a list of tasks to be carried out). A steering committee is appointed for the project. For larger or more complex projects, the committee will meet monthly or weekly. Communication is less formal for small, uncomplicated projects, where the PM would stay in touch using e-mail, telephone, or face-to-face conversation.

Clarity and Management Reporting

The PMO uses the Clarity project and portfolio management software from Computer Associates. Clarity is an enterprise product (rather than one that just resides on individual PCs) and is maintained on FCG's servers. The project plan is maintained on Clarity. First Consulting Group staff enter their hours into Clarity weekly, and a list of issues and risks for each project is maintained. Microsoft Outlook is still used extensively to communicate about the project.

A dashboard report (figure CS1-2) for all active projects is distributed monthly via e-mail as a PDF attachment and is also on an online portal. It shows, using green and red icons, whether a project is on time and on budget. Reports for individual projects (figure CS1-3) are prepared weekly by project managers and distributed via e-mail as a PDF attachment to the executive sponsor (a vice president who approved the project), the project sponsor (the operating manager who requested the project), and the project team doing the work. Chief information officer Marx would like to see the organization move to an even greater level of transparency. Sponsors should be able not

Figure CS1-2. Project Management Office Executive Dashboard

PMO Executive Dashboard

University Hospitals

| Week Ending | 9/22/2006 |

Project	Project Manager	Start	Finish	% Complete	Approved Budget	Exec. Sponsor	Project Sponsor	DIO	Overall Status	On Schedule	On Budget	Quality Status	Scope Status	Resource Status
Enterprise Oracle Document Management	BALUCH	10/10/05	11/24/06	91	574,534.00	Kevin Roberts	Michael Vehovec	Kelly, Mike	●	●	●	●	●	●
Project Assessment	The project is on schedule for migration from the test to production environment starting on the evening of 09/29 and go-live on 10/02/06.													
Topics For Management Discussion	No topics for management discussion.													
CMIS Patient Feed	BALUCH	06/06/05	09/29/06	95	49,280.00	Kevin Roberts	Matthew Love	Ciraldo, Lou	●	●	●	●	●	●
Project Assessment	The project is scheduled to close on 09/29.													
Topics For Management Discussion	No topics for management discussion.													
UHC Surgery System Implementation	BALUCH	07/15/04	01/02/07	64	2,105,500.00	Dr. Keating	Laurie Canala	Assenmacher, Amy	●	◇−◇	●	●	●	◇−◇
Project Assessment	The project schedule has slipped but we are working on resolving our nursing shortage for project work. We are currently working with Bedford administration to obtain nursing backfill resources that can free up current OR nursing time to work on the project.													
Topics For Management Discussion	The Soarian Project has an impact on our go-live plans. The current challenge relates to possibly revising our current system build approach to accommodate both a PB registration and Unity billing interface and/or also accommodating a Soarian implementation. At some point as we implement, the surgery system will need to support dual system environments - both front-end and back-end. The Soarian project will be adding significant complexity to our system build plan and we are working on meeting that challenge.													

Source: Reprinted with permission from University Hospitals, Cleveland, Ohio.

15

Figure CS1-3. Project Status Report

Project Status Report

Project	UHHS-TP-CMIS Patient Feed
Project Manager	BALUCH, JOHN
State	Active
Week Ending	09/22/2006

Project Description

This purpose of this project is to create and implement the interfaces necessary to load both Inpatient and Outpatient data feeds (Medical Records, Utilization and Payment Posting) into the CMIS - Clinical Cost Manager (CCM) module for Richmond Hospital.

Schedule

	Actual	Baseline	% Complete	Variance
Start	06/06/2005	06/06/2005	95	
Finish	09/29/2006	09/29/2006		0.00
				0.00

Status

Overall	●	Quality	●
Financial	●	Resource	●
Schedule	●	Scope	●

Project Assessment

The project is scheduled to close on 09/29.

Accomplishments This Period

IT&S ran a special query extract this week on one day's visits. Cyndee and Scott are to have reviewed and tested those patient records in Affinity against the query extracts. The purpose of the test is to validate that the balancing differences between Affinity reports and the query extract reports is due to patient type and visit type changes happending within Affinity and that the query extracts are only able to account for the final record.

Work Planned For Next Period

If the test is successful, then we will have a process to account for variances that happen on a weekly basis.

The project is scheduled to close on 09/29 based on sign-off from Matt Love.

Topics For Management Discussion

No topics for management discussion.

High Priority and Escalated Issues

Priority	Issue ID	Issue Name	Target Date	Assigned To
	002027	Outpatient balances do not balance to Affinity reports	9/12/2006	J. BALUCH

High Priority Risks

High	Risk ID	Risk Name	Target Date	Assigned To

No Risks.

Recent Change Requests

Change ID	Change Name	Target Date	Budget	Sched	Scope

No Change Requests.

Figure CS1-3. (Continued)

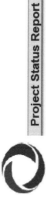

Project Status Report

Milestones - Next 90 Days

Milestone	Target Date	% Complete
Sign-Off on Weekly and Monthly file load process	9/22/2006	0
Project Completion	9/29/2006	100

Overdue Milestones

Milestone	Target Date	% Complete
Sign-Off on Weekly and Monthly file load process	9/22/2006	0
Final review / validation of weekly/monthly file loads	9/15/2006	0
August - Outpatient Monthly file load	9/8/2006	0
July - Outpatient Monthly file load	8/11/2006	0

Project Schedule

Phase	Actual Finish	Baseline Finish
Design	9/18/2006	9/18/2006
Test	8/10/2006	8/10/2006
Deploy	9/18/2006	9/18/2006
Conclude	9/29/2006	9/29/2006

Source: Reprinted with permission from University Hospitals, Cleveland, Ohio.

only to view dashboard reports but also to drill down and see as much detail as they want on Clarity.

Change Management

Changes in scope, timeline, and budget must be approved. Only changes within a budget category that balance out to the same amount do not require a change request. The PM completes the change request form and submits it to the PMO director for approval. A form is then circulated using Outlook and signed electronically. A change request (e.g., pushing back the "go live" date) must be signed by the executive sponsor, the project sponsor, the relevant DIO, and the PM. The project sponsor owns the budget and is the primary decision maker for changes in the budget. It is important for the PMO and the PMs to follow this process because FCG pays a financial penalty for missing a project end date.

Responsibilities and Accountability

The project sponsor presents the project to the IT advisory committee and the IT steering committee. University Hospitals has a "closed loop" governance process. If approved, the same sponsor must return six months to a year after the project goes operational to attend a meeting of the steering committee and present a report on the completed project that parallels the initial proposal (which is presented on one slide). A side-by-side comparison is presented of the cost, objectives, and start and end dates. Marx believes this procedure reinforces the idea that the project sponsor is accountable for making the project work: "It's a huge cultural shift. We're in the third year of the process, but it's happening. There's still a lot of finger pointing, but project sponsors know they have to come back. We also ask them what went very well and what didn't work so well to help others go through the process."

When a project is approved at an IT steering committee meeting, the CEO usually asks who "the person to hug" will be if the project succeeds and is on time and on budget. The project will not get approved unless the project sponsor agrees to be that person. The closed-loop process (i.e., from presentation of the proposal to presentation of closing results to a committee chaired by the CEO) makes it difficult for the sponsor to move responsibility to other parties, including IT staff. With the exception of infrastructure projects, for which the CIO is the sponsor, an operations sponsor is accountable for all projects. The lack of single accountability is viewed by Marx as an important reason that projects failed in the past. "Who should be singularly accountable for an application to run the OR? Can IT affect the processes within the OR? No. Can IT tell people in the OR how to use the application right? No. Who can? It's really the head nurse in the OR who is the project sponsor. She is singularly accountable. We can give them the hardware and software, but at the end of the day we can't tell them how to operate their business."

The project sponsor has high expectations that the PM will do the majority of the work. The PM must take the approved project scope or business plan and expand it to a project plan that includes critical details such as the actual start and end dates and the specific staff to be utilized. None of this can be determined earlier because the project has to move through the governance process first.

The annual meeting of the IT steering committee to approve projects for the following year does not result in the specification of the order in which projects will be done. The PMO director receives a list of projects approved for the coming year and must determine start and end dates for each project based on the priorities defined by the IT steering committee, the CIO, and DIOs as well as on the availability of project managers. The goals, risk, and alignment information provided by the DIOs are also being entered, beginning in 2007, into Clarity to create a score to be used in prioritization. It is expected that future use of Clarity's portfolio management module will help the prioritization process by presenting charts and tables that show the impact on staff of alternative start and end dates and documenting the dependencies involved in projects.

The PM has to work with the project sponsor, the DIO, and the functional managers of IT&S staff (e.g., programmers and database administrators) to determine what staff can be assigned or acquired for the project. The resources are defined in the project scope document, so functional managers are aware of what resources will be required, but not the start and end dates. The PM has to work with them to assign existing staff or to identify outside resources (e.g., consultants) to either work on the project or do the current work of staff assigned to the project.

If an outside vendor is involved, the PM is responsible for tracking the budget, seeing that invoices are paid, and working with the vendor to remove any roadblocks to the completion of the vendor's work, for example, delayed shipment of hardware.

The PM is responsible for identifying such issues and risks, communicating them to the project sponsor and working to mitigate them, regardless of whether an outside vendor is involved. Issues and risks are initially identified in the project scope document, and a list is maintained in Clarity that all project team members can access.

Once staff are assigned, the PM is responsible for contacting project staff to determine when tasks are completed. The PM is the facilitator and organizer of the project. If staff are not able to devote the time promised to the project or not able to do the work, it is the job of the PM to go to that person's manager and resolve the problem. First Consulting Group has service level agreements with UH that include completing projects on time and on budget (unless any change has been authorized) or, as mentioned earlier, paying a specific financial penalty.

This process differs significantly from one in which functional managers supervise staff directly to ensure that work is being carried out. Project managers do not manage the people; they manage the work. The PM, while not responsible for the annual review of particular staff, monitors when tasks are completed. However, they are not aware of all the work being done by each staff member and resource manager, which they need to consider when asking for resources. The executive sponsor, DIO, and project sponsor receive weekly status reports on progress. This could be described as a form of matrix management in which staff doing the work report to both a functional manager and the PM. However, PMs do not participate in formal human resources tasks, including performance review and recruitment.

The new governance and project management processes require a considerable change in the attitudes and behavior of operations staff. Projects involving computer hardware and software are no longer owned by IT&S, but by the business units. The PMO, however, is part of FCG, which pays penalties if projects are not completed according to agreed-upon dates. The PMO is responsible for ensuring that projects get done on time and on budget, but everyone, in theory, has an interest in actively participating and cooperating to make sure projects are successful.

Not all projects are managed by the PMO. Very large strategic projects, such as the $100 million EHR project, operate differently. Projects that are considered highly strategic and transformational tend to have dedicated project teams. While the project will be run outside of the PMO, there will be meetings with the PMO to ensure coordination. A PM, not part of the PMO, directly supervises dedicated staff in a more traditional management structure. Once the project is implemented, the project staff become operations staff and run the system. Skills and control are considerations in deciding whether the PMO should manage a project. Implementation of Enterprise Resource Planning software, for example, was run by the CFO at Case Medical Center in Cleveland because none of the PMs was believed to have the necessary skills. Thus, a physician and a nurse are the managers of the EHR initiative for the same reason. OneNet, the replacement of the entire network with one that uses Internet standards and allows for Voice over Internet Protocol calling, is another example of a project that was not managed by the PMO.

Value of Project Management

Chief executive officer Zenty believes the value of project management is the opportunity to "vet a project before it is accepted and the rigor of the analysis that is done from a business standpoint, from a process standpoint, from an expected outcomes standpoint, and an involvement standpoint." He does not believe that the end owners are as willing to "kick the tires" of an IT project as they are a construction project. The end users need to understand the capabilities and drawbacks of the system up front. They need to raise questions and not wait for a consultant or IT staff to tell them what they are and to find a solution. A project management office can identify the key issues in change management that a technology will require. How much time is spent on change management depends on the scale of the project.

Marx believes that UH has moved to a higher level of professional accountability. Projects are more likely to meet expectations. He is able to answer questions from executive staff because of the information maintained by the PMO using Clarity. For example, he was recently able to show the CEO where resource constraints would occur because of the implementation of the EHR. He was able to demonstrate how many full-time equivalents were available and how many would be needed. "When I showed them the data-driven graphics, there were no more questions."

Measuring Project Management Office Success

Zenty feels the PMO is successful because projects are completed. Marx quantifies that success rate, indicating that UH has improved its on-time and on-budget rate from 50 percent of projects ending on time and on budget to 90 percent today. Of course, projects may still continue to miss time and budget goals even with a PMO, as uncontrollable factors may arise. For example, a vendor may overstate what a system can do. The vendor might promise that the product will work in "all" environments, but it ends up failing to work in a particular hospital, making it necessary for the vendor to do development work that delays completion of the project. Another example is when a staff resource is pulled away from the project to deal with a critical situation. A programmer with expertise in an internally developed patient billing system, for instance, may be pulled away from a project when that system goes down. There may be no staff available to take the programmer's place, or someone with less knowledge may be called on to fill that role, resulting in delays.

Cost of the Project Management Office

Marx believes that UH is getting good value from its outsourced PMO. University Hospitals is getting trained and certified PMs and a good management tool (Clarity) that is maturing. He would not eliminate the PMO to reduce costs and go back to a 50 percent success rate.

All managers in every field spend time managing projects. The PMO provides staff trained in project management to take on those tasks, freeing operations staff and IT functional managers to do their other work. University Hospitals's accounting systems do not measure the time spent on project management, so savings from the reallocation of tasks cannot be measured. Current systems also do not measure the cost of inefficiency—for example, the time spent by a less experienced person in excess of what a trained PM would spend to effectively manage a project. On the other hand, the additional cost of the PMO is easy to measure and could be criticized as an "add on" cost that simply increases administrative costs.

The expectation is that project management carried out by trained professionals is more efficient and consistent. Monitoring task completion and the timeline, for example, is done frequently for all projects. A consistent methodology ensures that accurate information on project success, timelines, and budgets is collected on all projects. Using an existing methodology and templates (e.g., for a project scope document) can also avoid wasting the time of operations staff.

Zenty notes that he would not carry out a major construction project without an architect and engineer who can ask the right questions. Likewise, he would not take on a major IT project without someone trained in project management.

Portfolio Management

University Hospitals's project management process and PMO continue to develop. An important new component is the use of Clarity's portfolio management module. Information on new projects is being entered into Clarity, including projects for the coming year approved by the IT steering committee that are not active because start dates have not been set (projects are not currently entered until a start date is set and a PM is assigned). Additional information on active projects is also being added.

The benefits of using Clarity are both operational and strategic. On the operations level, having information on all projects will provide a picture of how staff resources are being used across all projects and what resources will be required in the future. Scenarios can be run in which the start and end dates of projects are changed to determine the effect on staff utilization, helping to clarify the interdependencies between projects. University Hospitals and the PMO will be able to move from being reactive to proactive in scheduling staff resources and determining project start and end dates.

Until portfolio management is implemented, there is no way to look across all projects to see how staff are being allocated. The PMO director keeps a spreadsheet that describes how PMs are allocated, but she has no way of seeing how other staff—for example, database administrators—are being allocated across all projects. Each functional manager is now asked whether staff are available. Currently it is possible, using Clarity, to see what percentage of an individual's time is being used, based on time sheets submitted, but not how all of his or her time was allocated in the project plans. With portfolio management, it will be possible to see who is overcommitted today, what the forecast is, as well as what the current staffing levels are in FCG's contract with UH.

Projects for the coming year that have been approved by the IT steering committee must be scheduled while taking into consideration the portfolio of existing projects yet to be completed, including the 28 percent (in 2007) of active projects that were not planned at the beginning of the year. There are many alternative scenarios for managing the new set of projects, but the choices are difficult to examine unless a complete view of all projects is available. It is hoped that using Clarity's portfolio management capability will make this process less complex.

On a strategic level, use of Clarity's portfolio management module will allow existing and new projects to be viewed in groups, according to their ranking on criteria related to their importance to and alignment with the strategic goals of the organization. These rankings are determined at the annual "big board" meeting, where projects for the coming year are approved. The DIOs are currently being asked to score projects on strategic alignment, complexity, and risk. These scores will be entered into Clarity and used to determine the start and end dates of projects. Executive management will be able to view the extent to which resources are being devoted, for example, to regulatory compliance as opposed to market expansion.

Sponsors want money approved for the current year to be spent by the end of the year because they are concerned that future funding would be reduced. Thus, pressure is felt to start projects immediately regardless of their importance to UH strategy. Portfolio management will give the CIO the information he needs to explain and enforce the prioritization of projects.

What Marx would like to be able to do in the future is to "drag and drop" projects in Clarity and view the changes in resources and the timeline that would occur. Clarity has the capability, and "we're six months away from that," according to Marx.

PART I

Estimating Benefits and Making the Business Case for Information Technology

Introduction

IN PART I, we focus on how benefits are estimated before making an investment in information technology (IT). Estimating benefits can help organizations move from a focus on technology to a focus on solving problems. Managers and clinicians are faced with choosing among numerous technologies that provide benefits that may or may not address problems facing the organization. Individuals in the organization may champion those technologies as the newest and best in the field. By estimating what benefits are provided related to actual problems facing the organization, the process of selecting technologies can be simplified. Such estimates also help to set realistic and explicit expectations, avoiding the disappointment that can occur when users discover that the benefits they thought could be achieved are not realized.

Estimating benefits requires considering the financial impact, process improvements, and intangible benefits of the investment. *Intangible benefits* are those that cannot easily be expressed in dollar terms, such as improved patient and staff satisfaction. A number of methods for conducting a benefits study are explained, as are methods for carrying out a financial analysis. The steps in creating a business plan to support a recommendation are then defined.

No consensus has been reached on the extent to which financial criteria should drive investment decisions. Some health care organizations will require a financial analysis that estimates return on investment (ROI), net present value, payback period, and other financial measures. Minimum values for these measures may be required before an investment is approved. Other organizations will conduct a financial analysis only to determine the magnitude of the financial commitment and risks involved. If capital is available, the decision to invest is based on the nonfinancial benefits that will result. These could include regulatory compliance, an increase in patient satisfaction, or competitive pressure. If the organization has developed a balanced scorecard, it may be used to assess the effect of the investment.

Is Defining Benefits Too Hard and Unreliable?

> **Projects can be placed into three categories: operational, tactical, and strategic. The complexity, expense, and difficulty involved in evaluating an IT investment vary according to the category it falls into.**

Enough stories are circulating about cost over-runs and elusive benefits to make managers skeptical about whether the costs and benefits of IT investments can be estimated. Before preparing a business case (or when presenting the results) it is important to recognize the differences among IT projects. Projects can be placed into three categories: operational, tactical, and strategic. The complexity, expense, and difficulty in evaluating an IT investment vary according to the category it falls into.

"The first category is strictly *operational;* it is a technological replacement for manual processes, either business or clinically related. There are benefits associated with the automation of these processes, primarily in cost reduction through improved efficiency, but also in terms of improved accuracy. These are fairly simple to evaluate using traditional financial management evaluation tools" (Boles and Cook 2005, 197).

Replacing a paper form with an online one is an example of an operational project. The cost of paper and printing is eliminated, as is the cost of moving, storing, and finding the form. If drop-down menus and restrictions on what can be entered are included, the accuracy of the data and the ease with which they can be collected and aggregated can also be improved. Information technology infrastructure projects are also operational. Examples are replacing a network and changing e-mail systems and servers.

"The second category, *tactical,* expands the business and clinical processes to include decision support. . . . This category of IT investment often requires a change in thinking and in the way of doing things. Thus, it is more difficult to implement, has a greater failure rate, provides important evaluation difficulties, and its benefits are more difficult to realize" (Boles and Cook 2005, 197).

Implementing computerized physician order entry (CPOE) is one way of replacing paper with online forms, but it also adds the capability of helping physicians by offering information (e.g., on drug interactions and patient characteristics that could affect ordering) and advice (e.g., on drug effectiveness). Reduction in errors and improved quality are usually cited as benefits, but determining the extent, value, and timing of those benefits is considerably more complex. Not all physicians will change their behavior immediately, and any change may occur over time. Baseline data must be collected to estimate the change resulting from CPOE. If patient outcome is selected as the measure of quality, the relationship between a change in ordering and final outcome has to be determined.

The third category is *strategic.* "Here, IT is considered to be an integral component of a product line. . . . IT has a role in the formation of the organization, how it develops, with whom it has relationships, how it delivers health services, and the extent to which it is a leader or follower, agent for change, innovator, or organization that lets others take an initial risk" (Boles and Cook 2005, 198).

Strategic projects can be identified by an analysis that identifies the strengths, weaknesses, opportunities, and threats facing an organization (Swayne, Duncan, and Ginter 2006, 285–88) or by an analysis of how a health care organization can attain or retain a competitive advantage (Wager, Lee, and Glaser 2005, 314–60). An example would be the establishment of a telemedicine program designed to serve a surrounding region or international patients. This could involve not just a few services (e.g., dermatology) but also a complete strategy of expanding the organization's mission. Boles and Cook (2005, 198) believe that an enterprise IT strategy "has the greatest potential for failure. . . . [I]t is expensive, is complex, and requires a different way of thinking on the part of all users."

Evaluation of tactical and strategic projects might at first seem easy. For example, the organization could determine if quality, volume, revenue, and profit expectations were met. Understanding what role the technology played, as opposed to the behavior of the users and stakeholders, is much more difficult. The Next-Care Urgent Care case study at the end of part I illustrates the difficulty of separating the effect of more than one initiative.

Thinking in terms of operational, tactical, and strategic categories of IT projects is useful in understanding the difficulty of creating and building confidence in a business case for a particular information technology. For some technologies, estimates of benefits and costs will present few challenges, while for others, skepticism about the numbers will remain even if the organization goes forward with the project. The seven steps to creating a successful business case, described at the end of part I, will help to prepare a business case that recognizes these differences.

Estimating significant positive benefits, of course, is not enough. In parts II and III of this book, we describe some of the tasks involved in effectively managing implementation and ensuring that benefits are actually received.

What All Hospitals Should Be Doing

1. Estimate the benefits of an IT project before implementation.

2. Reach agreement on the benefits—tangible and intangible, hard and soft—that are being used to justify the expenditure.

3. Decide on the dollar or effort threshold for writing business cases for IT investments and mandate business cases (recognizing that some projects are not evaluated by financial criteria).

4. Require executive sponsorship of IT projects. Projects with strong sponsorship are more likely to succeed.

Decisions

A number of decisions must be made by health care managers about estimating the benefits of IT projects and building a business case for them. The following questions help address the relevant issues.

Should we estimate benefits? Which benefits are essential, and which provide secondary support for the decision to invest? Estimating benefits in a way that addresses concerns about the validity of the results takes time and money. That money should be spent because the results are important. If an investment is being made primarily to improve patient care or to equal the progress of competitors, then a careful financial analysis of the benefits may not be needed.

Should we write a business case for IT projects? Which ones? Based on our experience, business cases for major IT investments are not routinely done. Some investments are considered necessary to meet regulatory compliance, to meet competitive pressures, or to meet the expectations of physicians and the board of directors. An electronic medical record (EMR) system is one example. It is important to define which investments require a business case, and why. For example, capital investments of more than $100,000 may require a business case when they are not needed for regulatory compliance nor are essential for another project already under way.

Many projects do not deliver the estimated benefits. How do we deal with this risk? An independent assessment of the likelihood that benefits will be received needs to be done. Who makes this assessment can vary according to the governance process in place, but it can be done by an internal advisory committee or by analysts in the finance department of larger organizations that specialize in IT projects. Clinicians can examine the expected benefits of clinical systems and assess how likely they are.

Do the chief executive officer (CEO) and chief operating officer (COO) need to be involved? When? Most major IT projects will succeed only if the units and departments that ask for them feel accountable for their success. None of these people report to the chief information officer; a clear signal needs to come from senior executives that they are interested and involved in the success of these projects. Leadership involvement can take the form of membership in IT or project steering committees or inclusion of project success in the personnel reviews that are conducted. The size of the organization and the size and critical nature of the project will suggest how personally involved the CEO and COO should be.

1

Estimating Benefits

To prepare a business case, measures must be selected that describe the effect that IT is likely to have. These measures can be categorized as (Cusack and Poon 2006, 6):

- Clinical outcomes measures
- Clinical process measures
- Provider adoption and attitudes measures
- Patient knowledge and attitudes measures
- Work flow impact measures
- Financial impact measures

Organizations will define some of these changes as "benefits" and will select specific measures to be used to support the investment. Measures will be selected because they directly relate to criteria that will be used to make the decision (see step two of chapter 3) and because measurement is feasible. Some of them will be defined as intangible because it is believed that they cannot be quantified in monetary terms. Intangibles include external requirements that do not have a dollar value. However, a reduction in the cost of meeting these requirements might be measured (Shekelle, Morton, and Keeler 2006, 14) through:

- Maintaining credentials
- Satisfying reporting requirements
- Satisfying a requirement to implement a quality improvement project
- Avoiding exposure to liability
- Building goodwill or reputation

Cusack and Poon's (2006) categories do not include market-oriented measures such as increased market share or improvement in consumer perceptions and intentions (a measure of competitive position). These benefits could be defined as intangible if a dollar value cannot be measured. Health care organizations can add measures that are related to their mission and strategies.

Examples of the benefits measures that could be selected appear in table 1-1.

Some organizations will find it difficult to convince clinicians to select measures that point out deficiencies in the care provided, even though it would help justify the investment in IT.

> **A major difficulty in estimating the benefits of health care IT is deciding whether to include just the benefits received by the funding organizations or those received by other individuals and organizations. A computerized medical record system might save physicians time and lower their medical liability risk, but should this be included in a determination of benefits? Or should the calculation only include benefits received by the health care organization that paid for it?**

Information on the benefits of health care IT will come from internal studies of current conditions (e.g., number of charts pulled, time between ordering and receiving a drug) or from published studies in other organizations, such as Partners HealthCare (http://www.partners.org) in Boston and Intermountain Healthcare in Salt Lake City, Utah (http://intermountainhealthcare.org).

> But these studies also have limitations, in terms of their usefulness to inform decisions about the adoption of . . . [health information technology (HIT)] elsewhere. The primary limitation is that these HIT systems were developed over the course of many years by technology champions at these institutions and, in a process of co-evolution, were adapted particularly to the working environment and culture of their respective institutions. Consequently, the "intervention" at these sites consists not only of the HIT system but also the local champions, who were often also the evaluators in published studies. Furthermore, it is challenging to calculate the

cost of the development of the HIT system as a whole, since this process occurred over many years at each institution. In addition, these systems are not commercially available from a vendor—and vendors supply most HIT systems in use in the U.S. (Shekelle, Morton, and Keeler 2006, 3)

The more functions and components the IT application has, the more serious these problems will be. For example, generalizing from the benefits received from a CPOE system with multiple decision support components would be more difficult than generalizing from the results of replacing films with digital images. It is important to define what CPOE means in terms of both functions performed and the extent to which it is used. The benefits of a CPOE system that allows residents to enter orders (but provides no help in making decisions) will be

Table 1-1. Examples of Benefits Measures

Clinical Outcomes	Preventable adverse drug events
	Length of stay
Clinical Process	Medication errors
	Number of orders given verbally
Provider Adoption and Attitudes	Percentage of orders entered by physicians on CPOE
	Use of help desk
Patient Knowledge and Attitudes	Patient knowledge of own medications
	Patient satisfaction
Work flow impact	Pharmacy callback rate (to gain information or resolve problems)
	Patient wait time in emergency department
Financial impact	Percentage of claims denied
	Cost of maintaining paper medical records

Source: Cusack and Poon (2006, 16–26).

dramatically lower than a CPOE system with decision support used by almost all physicians in the facility.

Two studies conducted at Partners HealthCare are described later in this chapter. Both can be used to suggest benefits measures and one methodology for data collection, but the extent to which the results can be generalized to other organizations is limited by the factors just described.

An analysis of published studies on health information technology costs and benefits was conducted in 2006 by RAND for the Agency for Healthcare Research and Quality (Shekelle, Morton, and Keeler 2006), and an interactive database of published articles is available online (see "Resources" at the end of part I). Of the 256 studies reviewed, 156 were about decision support, 84 were assessments of the EMR, and 30 were about CPOE.

Comparing Existing Technology to Alternatives— Should We Stay with What We Have?

Before investing in technology, it is important to consider whether benefits could be achieved by changing how work is done while remaining with existing technology. Implementation of IT is often part of a larger process of improving performance by examining how care is provided or administrative tasks are performed. Information technology implementation by itself can trigger reconsideration of how work is done that produces benefits. The extent to which benefits are produced by technology rather than other changes is not always easy to determine.

> **Before investing in technology, it is important to consider whether benefits could be achieved by changing how work is done while remaining with existing technology.**

For example, purchasing wireless phones to replace pagers may help house physicians and nurses communicate more quickly, but establishing and enforcing rules about the frequency of communication may also generate benefits. A new, formal process for the handoff of patients as shifts change may produce some of the benefits desired. Increased use of an existing EMR may lead to better documentation and a reduced need for phone calls.

NextCare Urgent Care (see case study at the end of part I) introduced a kiosk system, for patients to enter information themselves at registration, at the same time it expanded the number of lab tests done in-house and introduced a system for ranking and rewarding clinic staff for reducing wait times. NextCare chose to introduce the patient kiosks at the same time as these other changes rather than wait to see if the desired benefits could be achieved without the technology. This was in agreement with a company policy to pursue multiple initiatives at the same time during a growth period.

Technology can still be a good investment if it adds value, but that added value needs to be defined and estimated. For wireless phones, immediate communication could produce benefits that justify the cost. Similarly, the absence of an EMR for the near future may justify wireless voice communication because it results in reduced labor costs; fewer duplicative tests; and quicker, more effective care.

Financial Impact

The sources of information available on benefits include published studies, internal analyses, and expert opinion. The two examples that follow summarize published reports of internal studies of the dollar savings from implementing two technologies. While they are retrospective studies, the logic used could be applied to estimate future benefits.

Computerized Physician Order Entry at Brigham and Women's Hospital in Boston

Kaushal and colleagues (2006) estimated the benefits resulting from CPOE at Brigham and Women's Hospital (BWH) in Boston, part of Partners HealthCare, between 1993 and 2002.

Because the impact of the computerized decision support system (CDSS) at the hospital has been extensively studied, they chose to calculate the benefit of its components. The two components were renal dosing guidance and a clinical decision support tool to decrease the frequency of ceftriaxone:

1. "Renal dosing guidance saved the institution the most money [a cumulative savings of $6.3 million]. In this intervention, the system recommends drug-dosing adjustments based on the patient's renal function. In a large study of this intervention, the number of appropriate orders increased from 30% to 51% (p < 0.001) and mean adjusted length of stay decreased from 4.5 days in the control group to 4.3 days in the intervention group (p = 0.009). The annual cost savings were most heavily driven by the decreased length of stay" (Kaushal et al. 2006, 264).

2. A clinical decision support tool to decrease the frequency of ceftriaxone from twice a day to once a day was introduced in 1999, resulting in 80 percent of orders being switched to daily dosing. Kaushal et al. (2006) calculated a cost savings of $175,094 annually by multiplying the number of saved doses by the cost of each dose.

They distinguished between benefits that would be included in the hospital's operating budget and those that would not. The two previous examples would be included, but some work flow improvements "may not directly reduce operating costs since improvement in efficiency does not necessarily translate into full-time equivalent reduction" (Kaushal et al. 2006, 262–63).

They also noted the importance of prospective reimbursement in the magnitude of the benefits received. "If a patient's care is not prospectively reimbursed, then savings do not necessarily accrue to the hospital from an avoided [adverse drug event (ADE)] or an unnecessary test since the hospital may be reimbursed by the insurance company regardless of whether the utilization was avoidable" (Kaushal et al. 2006, 263). The hospital's average prospective payment during the study period was 80 percent.

Kaushal and colleagues estimated that the CPOE system operating for eleven years resulted in a cumulative net benefit of $16.7 million ($2.2 million annualized). The operating budget savings were $9.5 million ($1.3 million annualized).[1] They noted that it took more than five years for BWH to begin accruing a net benefit and more than seven years to begin accruing an operating budget benefit. The level and type of decision support were directly related to the amount of savings, and the majority of savings came from a relatively small number of the components of decision support. This led Kaushal and colleagues to recommend that hospitals focus on those components that increase the profitability of their CPOE systems.

They also noted that "less direct benefits of CPOE such as averted malpractice litigation from fewer ADEs" were not included. They further pointed out that the model "is purely cost avoidance and does not directly address increased revenue. CPOE systems often result in improved billing, but these savings were not incorporated in our benefit estimates" (Kaushal et al. 2006, 265).

The cost of the time devoted by clinicians and researchers in developing clinical rules was not included, but Kaushal et al. (2006, 265) believed these "hidden costs were piecemeal over many years and probably represented a relatively small part of the entire costs."

They also noted that realizing these savings is not automatic. "To achieve the types of benefits modeled based on BWH data, a hospital must have nearly 100% physician use, well designed CDSS elements, and effective interfaces among CPOE, pharmacy, laboratory, and medication administration record systems. Some hospitals have overcome large financial barriers to implement CPOE, only to fail to achieve widespread use due to physician resistance. In addition, the automated knowledge necessary for CDSS elements must be represented in ways that

---

[1]All results are present value figures reported in constant 2002 dollars. See the "Discounting, Annualization, and Constant Dollars" section below.

allow it to be readily interchanged between different computer systems" (Kaushal et al. 2006, 265).

Electronic Medical Records in Primary Care

Wang and colleagues (2003) estimated the net benefit of an EMR in a primary care setting using data collected from several internal medicine clinics at Partners HealthCare, published studies, and expert opinion. The estimated net benefit for a five-year period was $86,000 per provider (Wang et al. 2003, 397). When data were not available, expert opinion was obtained using a modified Delphi technique to arrive at group consensus with a seven-member expert panel.

Wang et al. (2003) constructed a hypothetical primary care provider patient panel using average statistics from Partners. This panel included 2,500 patients, 75 percent of whom were under 65 years of age; 17 percent of patients under 65 belonged to capitated plans. They carried out sensitivity analyses in which panel size was varied from 2,000 to 3,000 patients, and the proportion of patients under 65 whose cases were capitated was varied from 0 percent to 28.7 percent.

Costs were categorized as either system costs or "induced costs"—that is, those involved in the transition from a paper to an electronic system, such as the temporary decrease in provider productivity after implementation. "Based on our experience, we modeled the induced costs of temporary loss of productivity using a decreasing stepwise approach, assuming an initial productivity loss of 20% in the first month, 10% in the second month, and 5% in the third month, with a subsequent return to baseline productivity levels. Using the average annual provider revenues for our model patient panel, this amounted to a revenue loss of $11,200 in the first year" (Wang et al. 2003, 398).

Financial benefits included were "averted costs" and increased revenues. Averted costs due to decreased utilization provide a benefit to providers for capitated patients. The benefits for fee-for-service patients are the result of charge capture and a reduction in billing errors (table 1-2).

Table 1-2. Annual Expenditures per Provider before Electronic Medical Record System Implementation and Expected Savings

	Annual Expenditures before Implementation		Expected Savings after Implementation		
	Amount	Reference	Base Case Estimated Savings	Sensitivity Analysis (Range)	Reference
Payer Independent					
Chart pulls	$5 (per chart)	*	600 charts	300–1,200	*
Transcription	$9,600	*	28%	20%–100%	*, 32
Capitated Patients					
Adverse drug events	$6,500	33–36	34%	10%–70%	‡
Drug utilization	$109,000	†	15%	5%–25%	‡
Laboratory utilization	$27,600	†	8.8%	0%–13%	37–39
Radiology utilization	$59,100	†	14%	5%–20%	‡
Fee-for-Service Patients					
Charge capture	$383,100	†	2% (increase)	1.5%–5%	25, 40
Billing errors	$9,700	†	78%	35%–95%	‡

* Primary data from the Partners HealthCare Electronic Medical Record System, Boston, Massachusetts.
† From the Department of Finance, Brigham and Women's Hospital, Partners HealthCare System.
‡ Expert panel consensus.
Source: Reprinted from Wang et al. 2003, copyright © 2003, with permission from Elsevier.

The average annual expenditures for a primary care provider before implementation of an electronic medical record was multiplied by the estimated percentage cost savings after implementation. This method for determining averted costs does not measure true marginal costs or the money the organization actually did not spend. Again, average annual expenditures before implementation and estimated percentage cost savings were determined by primary data collected from Partners's electronic medical record system, from other published studies, and from expert opinion.

Wang et al. (2003, 397) assumed a phased implementation, in which only basic electronic medical record features were available in the first years (e.g., medication-related decision support), and more advanced features were added in subsequent years (e.g., laboratory, radiology, and billing benefits) (table 1-3).

Sensitivity Analysis

Wang and colleagues conducted three types of sensitivity analysis to determine how their estimates would be affected by the assumptions they were making. Table 1-2 shows the ranges they used to recalculate the expected savings. A similar analysis was done for costs. For example, the number of chart pulls that would no longer occur was allowed to vary from 300 to 1,200, which would result in both lower and higher savings.

This analysis showed that the results were most sensitive to variations in the proportion of patients in capitated health plans because the net benefit varied from $8,400 to $140,100. The model was least sensitive to variations in laboratory savings, where the net benefit ranged from $82,500 to $88,300.

A "two way" sensitivity analysis was also performed using all combinations of the five most important variables identified in the one-way sensitivity analysis, and with combinations of one benefit variable with each of the three primary cost variables (software, hardware, and support).

Table 1-3. Five-Year Return on Investment for Electronic Medical Record System Implementation

	Initial Cost	Year 1	Year 2	Year 3	Year 4	Year 5	Total
Costs							
Software license (annual)	$1,600	$1,600	$1,600	$1,600	$1,600	$1,600	
Implementation	$3,400						
Support	$1,500	$1,500	$1,500	$1,500	$1,500	$1,500	
Hardware (refresh every 3 years)	$6,600			$6,600			
Productivity loss		$11,200					
Annual costs	$13,100	$14,300	$3,100	$9,700	$3,100	$3,100	$46,400
Present value of annual costs*	$13,100	$13,619	$2,812	$8,379	$2,550	$2,429	$42,900
Benefits							
Chart pull savings		$3,000	$3,000	$3,000	$3,000	$3,000	
Transcription savings		$2,700	$2,700	$2,700	$2,700	$2,700	
Prevention of adverse drug events			$2,200	$2,200	$2,200	$2,200	
Drug savings			$16,400	$16,400	$16,400	$16,400	
Laboratory savings					$2,400	$2,400	
Radiology savings					$8,300	$8,300	
Charge capture improvement					$7,700	$7,700	
Billing error decrease					$7,600	$7,600	
Annual benefits		$5,700	$24,300	$24,300	$50,300	$50,300	$154,900
Present value of annual benefits*		$5,429	$22,041	$20,991	$41,382	$39,411	$129,300
Net benefit (cost)	$(13,100)	$(8,600)	$21,200	$14,600	$47,200	$47,200	$108,500
Present value of net benefit (cost)*	$(13,100)	$(8,190)	$19,229	$12,612	$38,832	$36,982	$86,400

* Assumes a 5% discount rate.

Source: Reprinted from Wang et al. 2003, copyright © 2003, with permission from Elsevier.

A five-way sensitivity analysis was performed using the most and least favorable conditions for the five variables. When the most pessimistic assumptions were made, the model showed a net cost of $2,300 per provider. When the most optimistic assumptions were used, this analysis yielded a net benefit of $330,900 per provider.

The time horizon was also varied from two to ten years. When the time horizon was reduced to two years instead of five years, the net cost was $2,100 per provider, and when the time horizon was lengthened to ten years, the net benefit was $237,300 per provider.

Wang et al. (2003, 401) concluded that "the net financial return to a health care organization from using an ambulatory electronic medical record system is positive across a wide range of assumptions. The primary areas of benefit are from reductions in drug expenditures, improved utilization of radiology tests, improvements in charge capture, and decreased billing errors. Benefits increase as more features are used and as the time horizon is lengthened. In sensitivity analyses, the net return was positive except when the most pessimistic assumptions were used."

Process Improvements

A range of improvements can result from IT applications. Schmitt and Wofford (2002) report on a study of EMR implementation at Virginia Mason Medical Center, estimating the benefits that would result from components of the EMR. Table 1-4 provides their estimate of the savings in time and, eventually, full-time equivalents (FTEs) from the implementation of CPOE. They emphasize, however, that the benefits are not automatic. "A cost-benefit study will benefit a health care organization only if it follows through with a focused effort to realize the projected benefits. Implementation of an EMR requires a strong, organization wide commitment" (Schmitt and Wofford 2002, 56). Reductions in FTEs may not occur unless they are mandated by management.

On the other hand, improvements in quality and productivity could occur when the time required to complete a task is reduced. Managers need to decide if those improvements should be listed as benefits in place of some or all of the staff reductions.

While reductions in staff may not be possible, this does not mean that saving time does not produce dollar benefits. As one chief financial officer (CFO) describes, "However, we knew these efficiencies were not going to equate to a direct reduction in the work force. In reality, you're not going to lay off nurses, but redeploy them. In other words, some of the time the nurses spent doing documentation would now be devoted to patient care, so the nurses would have the capacity to care for more

Table 1-4. Benefits from Electronic Medical Record System Implementation at Virginia Mason Medical Center

Benefit Provided by the EMR	Methodology and Assumptions Used in Estimating Benefit	Eventual Dollar Benefit (Annual)
Laboratory and Radiology Order Entry		
Reduction in time spent managing laboratory and radiology orders	Hospital unit staff and certain clinic staff spend on average 11% of their time processing orders. Approximately 35% of this labor could be translated to staffing reductions, saving roughly 24 full-time equivalents (FTEs).	$921,044
Reduction in laboratory/ radiology FTEs needed to process orders	Currently one laboratory FTE and two radiology FTEs are dedicated to processing orders. These positions could be eliminated.	$93,600
Reduction in laboratory FTEs involved in working suspended charges	Two FTEs currently are dedicated to working suspended charges. These positions could be eliminated.	$62,400

Source: Schmitt and Wofford (2002). Reprinted with permission.

patients. Such changes in care delivery had derivative savings potential. It might mean reducing the amount of recruitment needed to try to find nurses to fill vacancies, since turnover would likely decrease as nurses felt more satisfied with how their time would be spent. This would also mean we could decrease our level of dependence on agency nursing—which is not only costly but less effective than having our own staff" (Healthcare Financial Management Association and Cerner 2005, 4).

Intangible Benefits

Keen and Digrius (2003, 45) believe that "tangibility is an opinion adopted by a group, not an absolute." The following case, provided by the U.S. Government Accountability Office (2003), illustrates how tangibility could vary.

Danville Regional Medical Center

Danville is a 350-bed, private, not-for-profit community hospital serving a rural population. It implemented a medical administration check (MAC) application as one component of its EMR system. The MAC utilizes bar-code technology and wireless scanners to provide positive identification of drugs and patients at the point of care. Patients' bracelets, all medications, and nurses' identification badges are bar coded; no inpatient receives medication without bar-code verification technology. Bar-code technology is integrated into a wireless network and EMR. Patients' charts are updated when medication is administered. Reported cost and cost-related benefits were as follows, according to the U.S. Government Accountability Office (2003):

- Prevented 1,241 wrong drugs or dosages, amounting to a $732,909 value in errors prevented (2002). (Only 17 percent were considered clinically significant.) A cost of $3,474 per ADE was assumed, based on Sublett's (2005, 26) averaging of values reported in Bates et al. (1997) and Classen et al. (1997), $4,685 and $2,262, respectively.

- Prevented 1,968 early or extra doses, amounting to a $116,226 value in prevented errors (i.e., potential over-doses) (2002). (Only 1.7 percent were considered clinically significant.) Again, a cost of $3,474 per ADE was assumed (Sublett 2005, 26).

Other reported benefits were:

- 50 percent decrease in phone calls to the pharmacy per day
- Increased patient safety
- Decreased medication errors
- Improved communication and documentation
- No paper charting required when medications are administered

This example illustrates that health care organizations make choices about what they feel are tangible and intangible benefits. A 50 percent decrease in phone calls could be a tangible benefit if the hospital was able and willing to determine the dollar value of the decreased time required. Danville chose to report data for two types of medication errors, but it recognizes that other types of error could also be reduced. Improved communication and documentation, as well as reduced paper charting, can also result in reduced labor and therefore lower costs.

In addition, Danville chose to use a published report rather than internal data in determining the cost of wrong drugs or dosages and early or extra doses. Although the published studies report results from a larger academic medical center, the assumption is being made that costs will be similar. In the absence of internal data or the resources to collect them, this assumption may be considered reasonable by managers. An alternative would be to use a range of costs in estimating the total benefit to examine the sensitivity of the results to this assumption.

Some benefits are frequently labeled intangible because they are difficult or expensive to measure, although current data systems can be used to provide measures that are closely related. One example is improved customer satisfaction. "In terms of measuring, most people would probably suggest a satisfaction survey. . . . While a survey would be useful, many key indicators of customer satisfaction can be extracted from most transaction-processing systems" (Murphy 2002, 109).

For health care, such indicators might include waiting time in the emergency department (ED) and length of time to receive the report of a lab test. A survey could initially be used to determine what factors patients consider important. To meet our definition of tangible, a dollar value would need to be placed on patient satisfaction, but the indicators can help us understand which groups of patients are likely to be satisfied or dissatisfied so their behavior and its financial consequences can be more easily isolated.

The Healthcare Financial Management Association and Cerner (2005, 3) offer this perspective on customer satisfaction as a benefit: "Include satisfaction. As you begin to knock down process barriers and improve the quality or amount of time physicians and nurses spend with patients, be sure to track customer service metrics. As an example, quicker response times in the emergency department stemming from efficiency in documentation may lead to fewer diversions, improved scheduling, and faster admission for patients on arrival. These changes are likely to create tangible improvements in customer and physician satisfaction."

Doing a Benefits Study

An estimate of the benefits that are likely to result from implementing a technology can be primarily based on internal studies and judgment or on external sources such as other facilities or published studies.

Internal Sources

Data on current costs and revenues can be collected from existing internal sources. Staff can then be asked to identify potential benefits. Using staff estimates and current costs, financial impact can be projected. For example, existing data could be used to determine the number of physician reports transcribed. Staff judgment can be tapped to estimate the rate at which physicians would switch to using voice-recognition technology for transcription. Estimates of the savings from not sending reports out for transcription over the next three years can then be made.

The advantages of this approach are that managers can (Jantos 2005, 7):

- Achieve buy-in and participation from as many individuals as necessary.
- Have individuals identify the benefits and hold them accountable for achieving them (in theory).
- Provide an expectation for implementation.

The disadvantages are that (Jantos 2005, 7):

- Assumptions may not be realistic.
- There may be undue pressure to identify benefits (area by area).
- The internal source approach may take a long time.

External Sources

Data on current costs and revenues can be collected by seeking out other facilities, vendors, and published sources. The same sources can be used to estimate benefits. Financial impact can then be calculated by applying those external numbers to internal data. For example, an estimate that 30 percent of physicians would be willing to switch to voice recognition technology could be applied to the current number of physicians and the number of transcriptions per physician.

Using external sources has a number of advantages. Other organizations may have had more experience with the technology and/or more resources to conduct a rigorous study of costs and benefits. This information can be collected quickly from publications and contacts with other organizations. A major disadvantage is that external data may be hard to generalize to another organization for the reasons described earlier (Shekelle, Morton, and Keeler 2006, 3). The buy-in and participation, accountability, and expectation for implementation that were identified as advantages of using internal data may also be missing.

Modeling

Another alternative is to combine internal and external data to simulate or "model" what is likely to happen. One example is the study undertaken by Wang et al. (2003), described earlier.

The advantage of this approach is that neither internal nor external data alone may reflect what managers believe will happen. By combining data and performing a sensitivity analysis, managers are able to develop estimates that reflect their own judgments. Using ranges rather than point estimates (e.g., between 20 and 30 percent of physicians will use voice recognition technology) allows managers to consider the impact of changes in the assumptions being made. Buy-in and participation, accountability, and expectation for implementation may result from involving staff in deciding on the data and assumptions to be used.

Process Mapping

An internal study of potential benefits could include process mapping to identify how work flows might be changed using IT to improve efficiency and effectiveness. Process mapping is a technique that will be familiar to professionals who have carried out a performance improvement project (e.g., as part of a continuous quality improvement, total quality management, or Six Sigma project). Process mapping involves observing and then creating a flowchart of activities.

Process mapping was part of the cost-benefit analysis undertaken by M.D. Anderson Cancer Center before implementation of its computerized patient record (CPR). "In these process-mapping sessions, multidisciplinary teams of care givers, business office staff, and support staff charted the flow of work activities. Process mapping was used at M.D. Anderson to identify problems in information 'hand-offs' and duplication of effort, as well as to begin understanding how a CPR could perform and change work processes. The findings of process mapping were integrated into department-specific questionnaires about how the CPR could streamline operations, improve quality, and lower costs. Detailed spreadsheets were created to show potential cost savings for various steps in each department's work processes" (Kian et al. 1995, 60).

Assessing Benefits during Implementation

Studying the benefits to be obtained can be useful even after the decision to invest has been made. Mohr and Ferguson (2005, 10) call this an "impact analysis."

> Once the decision has been made to implement, it may be easier to simply proceed without the additional work of performing an impact analysis. However, there are several ways an impact analysis can add value to an implementation. Before a full implementation, impact analyses can:
> - Provide departments with an understanding of future impacts/benefit of the implementation, as well as an expectation of what to expect with the implementation. This allows departments to make operational plans, such as adjusting staffing resources.
> - Identify weaknesses in an implementation and suggest special needs to make the implementation successful. For instance, the analysis may suggest additional training or communication to improve the success of the implementation.
> - Help distinguish implementations that provide the most value to the organization. These results can help to prioritize which projects to implement to maximize the value to the organization. Additionally, impact analyses require resources and performing implementations prior to an implementation can help identify which projects are worth the resources to analyze.
> - Provide post-implementation estimates so the success of the project can be evaluated.

Pilot projects can be used to estimate impact.

To obtain these benefits during implementation, a pilot project can be launched and studied and the results used in the rest of the implementation. "Pilots are very useful to provide insight into how a full implementation will 'work.' Pilots can also be used to estimate impacts and then use those results to apply to the full population" (Mohr and Ferguson 2005, 14).

Mohr and Ferguson (2005, 17) give the example of the elimination of printing electronic clinical notes for permanent storage in the paper medical record. Notes were being dictated, transcribed, and then printed, although an electronic copy was created during transcription.

> The evaluation team followed the following key steps or methodologies when performing the impact analysis for this project.
> - Pilot: Identified four representative study areas to collect data
> - Process Analysis: Developed process maps of current and future/Best Practice Note printing process
> - Process Analysis: Performed comparative analysis between current and future processes to identify quantitative and qualitative impacts
> - Data Collection: Observed and gathered data on current state of process
> - Data analysis: Determined quantitative changes to process and estimated projected impacts for study areas
> - Extrapolation: Extrapolated estimated impacts to all outpatient areas based on current Note volumes
> - Project Validation: Validated that impacts projected were achieved

The impact study showed that eliminating printing (Mohr and Ferguson 2005, 21):

- Reduced process steps from more than sixteen to seven
- Reduced the cost per note from $1.43 to $0.96
  - Estimated annual staff savings of 24 FTEs at approximately $1.2 million (validated one year later)

—Estimated annual supply savings of $500,000

- Increased patient safety by eliminating redundant paper copy of electronic note
- Eliminated backlog of filing paper notes

Asking physicians and other clinicians to consult an electronic note rather than a paper record is not a trivial request. It requires a change in how clinicians carry out their work during a medical encounter. By identifying the benefits during a pilot, the assumptions made in the original proposal can be partly validated before extrapolating benefits to the entire organization, helping clinical managers win support for the change.

2

Financial Analysis

FINANCIAL ANALYSES conducted for an IT investment can range from simple to complex. At the simpler end of the range, IT staff may simply identify the major costs of a current system and identify significant savings that would result from a new technology. For example, eliminating films with a picture archiving and communications system (PACS) in a radiology department eliminates the cost of paper, chemicals, and processing. The significant labor costs of storing and retrieving films are also avoided.

A more detailed analysis might determine productivity and revenue increases that might result. For digital storage of films using a PACS, the wait times for locating and moving films would be eliminated, which may mean that patients are seen faster in the emergency department or are discharged earlier. If a hospital is operating at capacity, earlier discharges allow more patients to be admitted and increase revenue. Earlier discharge results in higher net revenue under prospective payment. Because multiple physicians can use the same films without waiting, their productivity could also increase.

An analysis at the more complex and difficult end of the range might examine how immediate access to an historical archive of images affects patient outcome and what cost and revenue implications this effect might have for the hospital. The ability to locate films may also improve billing and reduce malpractice expenses.

How much time and money is spent on financial analysis will be determined by the magnitude of the expense, the perceived nonfinancial benefits of the technology, the need to adopt the technology to compete in a market, and the management style of both the board and senior management. For some organizations, particularly large academic medical centers, the board and senior management may quickly agree on the need to adopt a PACS after they are confident about the cost and the savings associated with getting rid of films.

> **Include an individual from the finance or financial planning department in the project review team to increase credibility and ensure accuracy.**

For other technologies, consensus may be harder to reach and a more complex financial analysis may be requested. For example, a "portal" that allows patients to schedule services and communicate with providers may meet with greater skepticism. The internal costs avoided are harder to identify because they are primarily labor costs, and reducing staff may not be viewed as a realizable benefit. Agreement needs to be reached on such labor reductions and other benefits estimated, for example, a reduction in no-show patients resulting from online communication. Information technology managers may also want to reach out to other organizations that have adopted the technology to obtain information on costs and benefits.

Taking the time to determine benefits can be useful for other reasons. "Soliciting widespread staff participation in assessing ROI paves the way for future acceptance of the technologies purchased" (Baldwin 2000, 56). For example, staff who have participated in flowcharting a manual process to determine how a computer application would streamline work flow are more likely to understand the benefits of the application. They may also more easily tolerate decreases in productivity during the implementation period. "Many physicians overlook the expense of paper chart retrieval. . . . They have staffs that become very adept at keeping the charts available. . . . They don't always appreciate what is going on behind the scenes" (Baldwin 2000, 64).

While a definition of the costs to be incurred will always be important, organizations will differ widely in how much time and money they want to invest in defining tangible benefits.

> "In the end, it's not hard dollars so much as strategic significance that will guide most business cases for [electronic health record] adoption. Rather than focusing on costs associated with acquiring the technology, discussions begin to center on opportunity costs associated with postponing investment" (Healthcare Financial Management Association and Cerner 2005, 4).

Financial Analysis Tools

The Healthcare Financial Management Association and Cerner (2005, 4) contend that "in the end, it's not hard dollars so much as strategic significance that will guide most business cases for [electronic health record] adoption. Rather than focusing on costs associated with acquiring the technology, discussions begin to center on opportunity costs associated with postponing investment." If the organization is unwilling to completely accept that opinion, then an analysis that includes benefits will be undertaken. There are a number of widely used tools for examining both costs and benefits to make an investment decision. Their advantages and disadvantages are described in this section.

Return on Investment

Boles and Cook (2005, 209) propose that ROI has been used in two different ways in the IT literature. "First, it has been used as a catch-all term to include all generic forms of return on an investment . . . internal rate of return, net present value (NPV), benefit-cost ratio, EVA, value at risk, and payback period. In this context ROI is an imprecise phrase without a specific definition. In the financial management literature. . . . Return on investment is calculated by dividing net benefits (benefits minus costs) by net investment. It provides an interest rate, or rate of return, that can then be compared with some benchmark or desired level."

Second, Boles and Cook (2005, 217) say, "The primary disadvantage of ROI is that it does not take into consideration the scale of the project. For example, one project may have a high ROI but be the result of a relatively small investment: a 50 percent ROI on a $100,000 investment will provide only $150,000 in benefits, whereas a 10 percent ROI on a $1,000,000 investment will provide $1,100,000 in benefits."

Another problem with calculating ROI by dividing net benefits by net investment is that it ignores the time value of money. While most IT projects involve a large cash investment in the beginning, benefits are received over time, requiring adjustments. The failure to make adjustments causes returns to be overstated (Finkler 2005, 197).

Discussions of ROI often assume that a single estimate has to be made before implementation. ROI can also be recalculated over time based on evidence from a pilot or partial implementation of the technology. "Data derived from initial programs will form the foundation of discussions with the board on furthering the organization's investment. Quantification and communication of success after the board's initial leap of faith is key" (Healthcare Financial Management Association and Cerner 2005, 3).

> The time value of money should be calculated in all ROI and benefit studies.

Time Value of Money

"In every case that a capital acquisition is considered, we must recognize that the acquisition is paid for either by borrowing money (and therefore paying interest) or by deciding not to invest the money elsewhere (and therefore failing to earn a return)" (Finkler 2005, 174). Time value of money (TVM) calculations, therefore, use compounding and discounting to determine the opportunity cost of capital investments (i.e., money that was not received because of the investment).

Assuming that an organization has $100,000 in the bank earning 6 percent interest, compounded annually, the total value at the end of two years would be $112,360. This includes interest on the 6 percent interest received at the end of the first year. This *compound interest* can be calculated using a pocket calculator or spreadsheet. Discounting is the reverse of compounding. If an organization expected to receive benefits worth $112,360 at the end of two years, that could be consider to be worth $100,000 today, assuming a *discount rate* of 6 percent. If benefits were less, a greater return could be obtained by simply depositing $100,000 in a bank. In this case, $100,000 would be the present value (PV) and $112,360 the future value (FV) of the investment. The formula for both are (Finkler 2005, 177):

$$FV = PV (1 + i)^N$$

$$PV = \frac{FV}{(1 + i)^N}$$

The interest or discount rate is i, and N is the number of years.

In calculating the benefits resulting from the CPOE system at Brigham and Women's Hospital in Boston, Kaushal and colleagues (2006, 263) "discounted all costs and benefits at a 7% annual percentage rate in accordance with the recommendations of the U.S. Office of Management and Budget for economic analyses performed for the federal government. This represents a societal discount rate rather than a hospital-specific rate."

The assumption here is that invested dollars would grow by an average of 7 percent per year, so the value of future dollars must be discounted using this rate before they are used to justify an investment. The discount rate is not intended to adjust for inflation but to recognize the cost of capital. While the discount rate could be increased to reflect inflation, this assumes that inflation affects all cash inflows and outflows equally. "A preferred method is to try to anticipate the impact of inflation on the various cash inflows and outflows and adjust each individual flow before calculating PV or FV" (Finkler 2005, 195). For example, competitive pressures may keep the cost of network services below the general level of inflation, while nurse shortages may be expected to result in higher increases than in the general labor market. A separate inflation rate should ideally be estimated for each, using past trends or expert opinion.

However, a single rate of inflation is frequently used instead. In calculating the benefits resulting from the CPOE system at Brigham and Women's Hospital in Boston, Kaushal and colleagues (2006, 263) took this approach: "All current dollar values for costs and benefits were converted to a constant dollar basis to adjust for inflation. We used the Bureau of Labor Statistics Producer Price Index time series for General Medical and Surgical Hospitals to deflate values to a constant 2002 base year."

A dollar received or spent in 1999 would be viewed as more valuable than one in 2002 because inflation has reduced the value of the 2002 dollar. Values for earlier years have been multiplied by an inflation factor so that they have the same value in 2002 dollars.

Net Present Value

Information technology investments require cash outflows and result in cash inflows. Organizations may also consider tangible benefits (those that can be expressed in money) as cash inflows in evaluating an investment. The NPV "approach calculates the PV of inflows and the PV of outflows and compares them. If the PV of the inflows exceeds the PV of the outflows, then the NPV is positive, and the project is considered to be a good investment from a financial perspective" (Finkler 2005, 190). Spreadsheets typically have an NPV function.

The discount rate could be set equivalent to the current rate of return on investments. It could also be set higher and serve as a *hurdle rate* or a *required rate of return*. Organizations may set hurdle rates to compensate for risk, believing that projects often do not yield the cash or benefits projected. For example, a discount rate of 10 percent can be set even if a hospital's cost of money is 8 percent (Finkler 2005, 190). This helps to account for risk. If no risks were evident, simply earning more than an organization could on alternative opportunities would be adequate. But if some risk exists that the expected returns from the project might not be realized, then it is important to have a hurdle rate that provides a reward if the project is successful, to offset the losses from unsuccessful projects.

Wang et al. (2003) calculated the NPV of an electronic medical record in a primary care setting. Table 1-3 in chapter 1 shows that the NPV per provider was calculated to be $86,400 over five years, using a discount rate of 5 percent. Cash inflows were included (e.g., from charge capture improvement) as well as cost reductions (e.g., transcription savings).

Murphy (2002, 33) cautions users of NPV in evaluating information technology infrastructure: "Accountancy-based techniques have a built-in bias against long-term investments because the longer it takes for the financial returns to be made, the lower the present value. Whereas this is correct in terms of the time-value of money, it tends to present potential investments in IT infrastructure in a relatively unfavorable light. This militates against the formulation of well-structured IT strategic planning, showing potentially crucial requirements such as infrastructure and security in an unfavorable light."

Internal Rate of Return

The NPV does not reveal what the actual rate of return on the investment was. "A small project with a 35 percent rate of return might have a lower NPV than a much larger project with a 12 percent rate of return" (Finkler 2005, 192). Some managers, therefore, calculate an internal rate of return (IRR) so that the rates of return of alternative investments are obvious. Information technology projects rarely have the same cash flow each year. While cash outflows may be the same (after the initial payment), cash inflows often vary because the benefits are received as components are implemented or as users are trained and utilize the components of a system. For example, physicians may begin entering drug orders, but a hospital may only gradually implement decision support tools that help reduce drug costs. "Generally, a computer program such as Excel or a sophisticated calculator is needed to determine the IRR with uneven cash flows" (Finkler 2005, 193).

Finkler cautions that the IRR technique assumes that future cash flows will be positive. If they are not, "the method produces multiple answers, and the actual rate of return becomes ambiguous. In such cases, one is better off relying on the NPV technique" (Finkler 2005, 194). In IT, this could happen if subsequent investments are made in upgrades that exceed benefits in a particular year.

Some investments are interdependent. It would not be possible to reject an investment in a network upgrade in order to install a PACS that requires such an upgrade even though the IRR of the PACS is higher.

Annualization

In determining the benefits resulting from the CPOE system at Brigham and Women's Hospital in Boston, Kaushal and colleagues (2006, 263) "calculated annualized values. Annualization converts the entire stream of discounted costs and benefits into a series of equal annual payments analogous to mortgage payments on a house."

Basing a decision on the cumulative costs and benefits of a project would ignore the length of time involved. We would value a $10 million net benefit received over two years differently from one received over five years. While discounting prevents overstating the value of future dollars, it does not provide an easily understood summary of the return. Some decision makers would prefer to know that a project will result in, say, "$1.3 million in annual operating budget savings" (Kaushal et al. 2006, 264) when comparing it to alternatives. Of course, annualization will mask the fact that the NPV of a project will typically be lower in earlier years because costs may be higher and benefits are received only as components are implemented and users are trained. Users could expect something close to $1.3 million in annual operating budget savings consistently.

Payback Period

The payback period defines how long it will take for the investment to be returned. An investment might have an ROI that meets a benchmark or desired level, but the payback period may be longer than an organization finds acceptable. This situation might be caused by the existence of risks (e.g., a change in reimbursement) that could make the forecasts for revenue or expenses less accurate over a longer period of time. A problem with using the payback technique is it "ignores everything that happens after the payback period. It also does not consider the time value of money" (Finkler 2005, 196). Projects that produce a higher NPV are ranked below projects that recoup their costs quickly. Using the payback period to decide between projects with similar returns may be one way to overcome this problem (Finkler 2005, 196).

Total Cost of Ownership

In order for a benefits study or ROI calculation to be valid, all of the costs associated with a project have to be tracked. These include hardware, software, network, and installation costs. Often forgotten or omitted are training and "backfill" costs (the cost of adding data from a previous manual or computerized system), increased staffing and training for help desk and desktop support people, software maintenance costs, and hardware replacement costs when it becomes obsolete. Often, these can add 25 to 50 percent to the cost of a project.

Table 1-3 in chapter 1 lists the costs reported by Wang and colleagues (2003) for the implementation of an EMR in a primary care setting. This example goes beyond what is typically shown in a business case by estimating the productivity loss during implementation. Such loss is one of the hidden costs that have led to the concept of "total cost of ownership." The idea is that the costs that appear on invoices and as line items in the IT or unit budget may not be all the costs incurred in implementation and operation.

For example, installation of a PACS may result in additional costs, such as (Briggs 2006):

- Integrating images and reports with other information systems within the hospital, at other facilities, and in physician offices
- Digital conversion costs for existing films
- Additional data storage capacity
- Upgrading networks
- Upgrading PCs and monitors
- Heating and cooling for an expanded data center

Adding a group of high-resolution PCs to allow viewing of images will result in additional call center requests and on-site maintenance by IT staff. These additional costs should be reported when a PACS is being considered (Dell Computer 2006):

Every organization that uses technology, no matter what size, can benefit by viewing IT expenditures from a Total Cost of Ownership perspective. This means looking beyond the costs of the end-user hardware, and considering other associated costs such as the following:

- Additional Capital Costs—software, IT support software and network infrastructure.
- Technical Support Costs—hardware and software deployment, help desk staffing, system maintenance.
- Administration Costs—financing, procurement, vendor management, user training, asset management.
- End-user Operations Costs—the costs incurred from downtime and in some cases, end users supporting other end users as opposed to IT technicians supporting them, which can be very costly.

This may require a change in accounting procedures. For example, the cost of procurement for project-specific hardware may not currently be determined. Staff may not even provide such data on time sheets, so an estimate or internal study may be needed.

Cost Estimation

Accurate cost estimation requires the determination of all the relevant cost elements (the total cost of ownership), data on the costs of prior implementations, and a cost accounting system that provides relevant data.

The organization needs to use both internal and external sources of information. If a project management office (PMO) exists, that unit (or a unit within finance) can collect information on the cost of implementation so that future estimates are improved. As noted above, the current cost accounting system may need to be changed to provide all the data needed to determine costs so that the data can be used in future implementations. This is particularly important in the implementation of applications with multiple components such as an EMR. Some hard-to-estimate costs, such as training, may be similar as each new component is rolled out. Peer organizations can also be a source of information on the cost of implementing particular technologies and vendor products. A data intelligence organization like Gartner Research (www.gartner.com) or Forrester Research (www.forrester.com) can also provide cost estimates for a fee or as part of an annual subscription.

Risk Assessment

Risks are threats to the success of a project. Risk assessment can be part of the prioritization process. Once a project is approved, risk management is one of the tasks involved in project management (see the appendix to part II). Risk can be quantified by creating a separate score and applying that to an estimate of net benefits.

A number of risk factors are at play in IT implementation (Benson, Bugnitz, and Walton 2004, 147):

- Project or organizational risk: the degree to which the success of the project depends on new or untested business skills or experience. This risk also considers the degree to which the business organization is capable of carrying out the changes required by the project.
- Definitional uncertainty: the degree to which the business requirements are well defined, well understood, and accurately translated into demand for information and application systems functionality.
- Technical uncertainty: the degree to which the project is dependent on untried technologies, and the degree to which the company possesses the appropriate experience in designing and building applications with the technology.
- Information systems (IS) infrastructure risk: the degree to which the technical environment possesses the required factors of data administration, communications, project management, and development.
- Technical risk: the degree to which the use of a particular technology requires new management, analytical, or developmental skills. The risk factor includes whether the requisite skills are available from the vendor or from the marketplace and whether training or new hires can provide the necessary technical expertise.
- Investment risk: the degree to which other, nonproject investments are required to make the project successful.
- Project management risk: the degree to which project managers are available and capable of dealing with the project's complexities, both technical and organizational.

Sicotte et al. (2006, 558) add to the list the following factors:

- Usability: Lack of perceived system ease of use. Lack of perceived system usefulness. Misalignment between system and local work practices (individual and interprofessional levels).

- Strategic and political: Misalignment of partners' objectives and stakes. Interorganizational conflicts. Power/political games.

Assessing all of these factors may at first seem complex and demanding. It is important to remember that stakeholders will be using these criteria even if they do not discuss them. Consider these typical objections to implementing CPOE:

- Project or organizational risk: "Physicians don't have the skill to use CPOE, and our IT staff isn't experienced in implementing clinical applications that affect the entire hospital."
- Definitional uncertainty: "Do we know what information physicians want and need?"
- Technical uncertainty: "A minority of hospitals have implemented CPOE; there are many vendors with competing products and our staff has no experience with them."
- IS infrastructure risk: "Our current IT infrastructure wasn't designed to support clinical applications throughout the hospital with 24/7 availability."
- Technical risk: "The current staff can't implement CPOE. Can we find the staff we need and depend on the vendor's support?"
- Investment risk: "CPOE requires work flow changes and staff training. Can we afford to pay for them?"
- Project management risk: "Our current staff has never implemented something this complex. Do we need a PMO to implement CPOE? Are we capable of developing an effective one, and can we afford it?"
- Usability risk: "It's going to take me two more minutes to order each drug. I usually just write the order in the chart and someone else enters the order. What do I get for the extra work?"

- Strategic and political risk: "CPOE helps the hospital and health plans control costs, but it costs me time, and who is going to pay me for that?"

So whether or not we formally consider the risks, they will be considered in the decision-making process. These risks certainly affect the pace of implementation of CPOE. A risk assessment can be conducted by creating a questionnaire that uses the definitions just provided and asks key stakeholders to rank the importance of each factor for a single project (on a scale of 1 to 5, for example). By compiling the data and discussing them, managers can gain an understanding of the attitudes and opinions of stakeholders like the board, medical staff, and senior managers. This may lead to a decision not to proceed or to formal efforts to deal with the risks through a risk management plan included in the project management process (see part II and particularly the appendix).

> **Whether or not we formally consider the risks, they will be considered in the decision-making process.**

Sensitivity Analysis

The Healthcare Financial Management Association and Cerner (2005, 3) recommend formally considering the risks when bringing a project to the board of directors: "Set ROI in a range. Boards feel more comfortable when there is a planned level of investment risk. Although it may be impossible to zero in on exact figures, setting ROI expectations based on most successful and least successful scenarios using reasonable assumptions will help dispel some concerns."

Sensitivity analysis is another method of incorporating assessments of risk into a calculation of costs and benefits. Partners HealthCare conducted such a sensitivity analysis for the implementation of an electronic medical record in a primary care setting (see the "Electronic Medical Records in Primary Care" section in chapter 1). Risk analysis assumes that single estimates are just that—estimates—and could turn out to be different from the projection. The question is what effect a different result will have on both costs and expected net benefits. For example, the analysis done by Wang et al. (2003, 400) showed that the results were most sensitive to variations in the proportion of patients in capitated health plans because the net benefit varied from $8,400 to $140,100. The model was least sensitive to variations in laboratory savings, where the net benefit ranged from $82,500 to $88,300.

Benefits Realization

> **It is important to realize that not having a formal benefits realization process raises the risk that benefits will not be received. This should be considered in setting discount rates and in carrying out a sensitivity analysis.**

Not all savings result in a change in the operating budget. Consider the impact of a CPOE system that was identified by a study at Montefiore Medical Center in New York. "The team found that nurses spent 4 to 6 percent of their work time on medication-ordering paper processes before CPOE implementation. After CPOE implementation, nurses saved about 20 minutes per day. At a savings of $14 per nurse per day, the time saved represented potential savings of $1,960 per day, or $715,400 per year" (Taylor, Manzo, and Sinnett 2002, 45).

The authors recognized that this "savings" would not "immediately accrue to the health care organization's bottom line." Nurses' freed time would instead "be directed towards patients and interventions to improve quality" (Taylor, Manzo, and Sinnett 2002, 46). If actual savings in labor costs are desired, a specific effort will have to be made to realize those savings, for example, by identifying in advance what positions would be eliminated when the system is fully operational. Ensuring that predicted dollar savings actually result in reductions in the operating budget is part of a process called *benefits realization.* This process will be discussed in greater detail in part III. It is important to realize, however, that not having a formal benefits realization process raises the risk that benefits will not be received. This condition should be considered in setting discount rates and in carrying out a sensitivity analysis.

> **When harvesting salary expense, entire positions have to be eliminated to have true cost savings. Saving a little time over a number of positions never results in cost reduction. These savings can be counted as efficiency improvements, which increase throughput and revenue, or as quality-of-care improvements due to additional time to accomplish the remaining tasks, resulting in fewer errors and improved job satisfaction.**

Project Ranking and Scoring

When projects are prioritized, the first ones on the list are usually those considered imperative by the organization (e.g., EMR in order to remain competitive, IT for a new building). Then come the projects required for regulatory issues. The Joint Commission may require, for example, that the hospital track how long it takes to wean patients off ventilators; HIPAA requires transmission of data in HL7 format. Next on the list are vendor-required upgrades. A vendor may indicate that it will no longer support an earlier version of its software. After that are projects that meet an ROI hurdle rate, such as payback in under three years. Finally come any other projects desired by a sponsor.

A capital budgeting process will require a comparison of projects other than those considered imperative or required by regulations. Organizations will differ in what factors are formally considered in making comparisons. They include strategic performance, compliance, financial impact, and risk. As discussed in this chapter, some organizations may set hurdle rates or minimum levels of return that are used to eliminate projects from consideration.

Other organizations will prefer a less rigid process that allows for the use of quantitative measures and professional judgment. University Hospitals (UH) (see the case study in the introduction to this book) has project sponsors prepare a one-page summary that describes capital and operating costs, expected benefits, and a rationale related to UH's strategy. A business case is required for projects more than $100,000. If approved by a senior vice president, the proposal goes to an IT steering committee. An annual meeting of the committee is charged with determining which projects will be included in the capital budget. Projects are rank ordered, and the cost of each project is added until a capital expenditure ceiling for that year is reached. This determines whether a project will go forward for the following year.

What is most important is to define a process that results in a commitment by senior management and project sponsors to support the project as the inevitable difficulties involved in implementation appear.

3

Creating a Business Case for a Major Information Technology Investment

> "Good ROI is more about conversations than calculations. More about psychology and politics than percentages. More about logic and wisdom than layers of numbers. More about the visibility of intangible (nonmonetary) benefits rather than obsessive focus on hard-money tangible payoffs" (Keen and Digrius 2003, xiv).

WHILE THE PROPONENTS of IT projects may believe that the need for the investment is obvious and imperative, technologies such as medication administration systems that utilize bar coding compete with other quality improvement investments. The decision may be when, not whether, to make the investment. One common tool to help senior management determine both value and priority is the business case. Organizations can decide when to write a business case, for example, when a project has estimated costs of more than $100,000—the criterion used by University Hospitals in Cleveland. If the project does not reach that threshold, a one- to two-page scope document can be written that simply states the costs and projected benefits. In this chapter we define what a good business case should contain.

It would be a mistake to view a business case as an irrefutable argument resting on financial calculations. Especially for tactical and strategic projects, doubt will remain on the reliability of forecasts and estimates. A business case is also aimed at people who have different interests and concerns. This is especially true in health care organizations, where professionals have different priorities. For example, a clinical department head may have an intense interest in IT projects that enable a new service but may have little concern for or understanding of why an upgrade of IT infrastructure, such as routers and servers, is needed to support new services. Health care professionals and consumers are focused on services and benefits, not IT:

> Financial ROI analysis for clinical system installations is incomplete in that it does not reflect the values of patients and health care professionals affected by the systems. From the perspective of the patient, the ROI is measured in safer and more effective medical care. Such care leads to better outcomes, better health, and higher levels of personal and professional productivity. . . . Similarly, the ROI measured by those who must make a capital investment is not the same as the ROI measured by health professionals who must take the time both to use CPOE systems and to adapt their work patterns to achieve the goal of improved quality of care. To the health care professional, the true ROI may be measured in terms of ease of use, total expended effort, and satisfaction with the results achieved. (Frisse 2006)

Keen and Digrius (2003, 273) describe a business case as "an analysis describing the business reasons why or why not specific investment options should be selected. A business case identifies the most relevant decision factors associated with a proposed investment, assesses their likelihood, and computes their value. Value includes both quantifiable and nonquantifiable considerations. The findings of the business case are then presented to the decision makers for their selection or rejection of the recommendations developed by the business case authors. The premise of a business case is that the investment option with the best cost-benefit payoff, related to all alternatives, should be selected."

A number of payoffs can result from improving the business cases that are developed for major IT investments (Keen and Digrius 2003, xiii):

- A higher likelihood that forecast project payoffs will, in fact, be realized or exceeded.

- Reduced political friction due to a shared sense that chosen investments are appropriate, objective, and fair. ("How come she got her project approved and we did not?")
- Decreased time and effort in evaluating and prioritizing projects for funding.
- Increased buy-in to management's investment decisions, due to a more open, objective, reliable process of selection and implementation.
- More confident and inspired ROI business case developers and sponsors.

Keen and Digrius suggest seven steps to creating successful business cases (figure 3-1).

Step One: Scope (Who Expects What?)

This step involves defining the business case contents and the project plan.

Task 1 is to define the business case drivers and project boundaries.

Business drivers are "major business factors that propel the need to make this decision now, rather than 6 months ago or 6 months from now" (Keen and Digrius 2003, 32). For health care IT, this could be regulatory compliance or the rapidly declining performance of critical components of the current IT infrastructure. If the drivers are not defined, the business case may not address issues of direct concern to senior management, resulting in rejection. Stating that the project would "improve the quality of care" is not enough. Saying that it would address a specific deficiency in a recent Joint Commission survey or offer comparable services to those recently started by an important competitor can increase the attractiveness of the project.

Boundaries identify exactly what is and is not included in this business case relative to (Keen and Digrius 2003, 33):

- Investment options to be assessed
- Span of the systems to be justified
- Organizational units involved in the value assessment

Figure 3-1.   Seven Steps Road Map to Creating Successful Business Cases

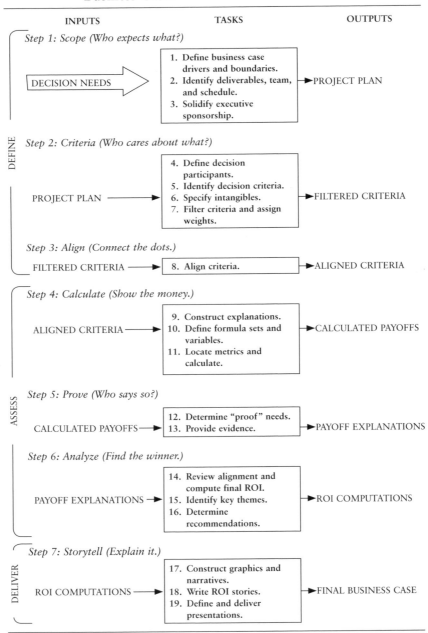

Source: Keen and Digrius (2003, 30). Reprinted with permission from John Wiley and Sons.

- Level of detail of the business case analysis and report
- People and resources to be consulted

In a business case for a new PACS, it would be important to state that the project will provide diagnostic quality displays for only radiologists, and only in specific buildings. The individuals to be consulted might be restricted based on expected use.

Task 2 is to identify the deliverables, team members, and schedule.

Task 3 is to solidify executive sponsorship.

> **"Any document that will influence senior management in making IT investment decisions requires an executive sponsor. This sponsor has overall responsibility to senior management for the quality and timeliness of the business case" (Keen and Digrius 2003, 34). Reaching agreement on, and getting commitment from, the executive sponsor is critically important.**

Solidifying could mean naming the executive sponsor of the project and when and how he or she will report to senior management. University Hospitals in Cleveland (see case study following the introduction to this book) requires an executive sponsor (a senior vice president) as well as a manager who will own the project. Both are expected to be present to report to the IT steering committee (which includes the CEO) when the project is being considered and six months after implementation.

Step Two: Criteria (Who Cares about What?)

"People embrace what they understand and care about" (Keen and Digrius 2003, 35). The purpose of this step is to "accurately determine the audience for the business case and the factors they will use (criteria) to make the investment decision" (Keen and Digrius 2003, 35).

Task 4 is to define who will directly influence or actually make the decision to invest.

Defining who will make the decision is the easier task. In health care organizations, many individuals can influence the decision while not formally being involved. This includes the clinical staff. The business case should formally recognize this wide group.

Task 5 is to determine the decision criteria that will be used to assess the value of the investment.

This may not be easy, as individuals may be unwilling or unable to articulate the factors they will use to make a decision. Three principles could be used to define criteria (Keen and Digrius 2003, 38):

- Business results focus: Defining value in terms of business results, not system features or functions
- "Who cares about what": Linking value to personal concerns of individual decision participants
- Alignment: Explicitly linking investment features to enterprise business needs

It would be simplistic and inaccurate to believe that the benefits described by the vendor and sponsors of a project are the primary concern of individuals involved in the decision. For example, physicians may be concerned about the effect of IT on the amount of time they have to spend caring for patients, a concern that will be shared by nursing staff. Managers may see the project as a drain on their budgets that is not compensated for with increases. These criteria need to be predicted and dealt with in the business case. For example, how will the organization deal with the need for nurses to spend additional time when a medication administration check system is introduced? Will additional staff be provided temporarily? Involvement and consultation are needed in order to predict the decision criteria that will be used.

Task 6 is to specify intangibles.

"Tangibility is an attribute indicating the extent decision participants believe a payoff can be quantified in monetary terms. . . . However, if they felt such savings could not legitimately be quantified, then the criterion would be classified as 'intangible'. . . . In the final analysis of business case work, tangibility is an opinion adopted by a group, not an absolute" (Keen and Digrius 2003, 45).

An increase in patient volume could be viewed as a tangible or intangible payoff from adopting a PACS. Decision makers might agree that a PACS delivers benefits that will be understood and valued by patients, who are then more likely to use the hospital. Or they could believe that patients make their decisions on the basis of unrelated factors, for example, the hospital where their physicians practice. This is not to suggest that intangible benefits are not important and should be excluded. Cumulatively, they may justify the investment.

The terms *hard benefits* and *soft benefits* are frequently used in discussing the benefits of IT. These terms are sometimes used as synonyms of *tangible* and *intangible,* respectively. Hard benefits are expressed in monetary terms and are, therefore, tangible. Our definition, however, is that hard benefits are those that are likely to be received, while soft benefits are considered less likely to be received. So even a tangible benefit, for example, a reduction in malpractice judgments, could be considered soft. While we can quantify the amounts of money paid in previous years for malpractice judgments, we may not feel that a reduction is likely to be achieved as a result of an IT project. While a PACS may result in fewer lost films, this may not result in lower malpractice judgments. The cause-and-effect relationship between lost films and lower malpractice judgments may not be accepted by decision makers. What is hard and soft is also a matter of opinion, and two managers can arrive at different decisions.

Hard-dollar savings are counted dollar for dollar against the cost of the project. A PACS project, for example, would include the cost of film and developer chemicals, the film library, and the cost of retaking lost films or films that did not develop properly as hard savings.

Savings accrued from malpractice suits that have to be settled because the films cannot be found, length of stay (LOS) reductions, or efficiency in not having to search for film are soft-dollar savings and are usually discounted. Some organizations may permit the inclusion of only part of a soft benefit to recognize that all the benefits may not be received. Typically they are counted at 25 to 50 percent of their apparent value. Thus, an organization might say that 20 percent of malpractice judgments (say, $6 million out of a total of $30 million) concerned lost films, but a reduction of only one-third of that amount ($2 million) can be included as a potential benefit of a PACS.

Having a benefits realization process in place might result in a higher estimate of the benefits to be received. A reduction in labor expenses because unit clerks have less paper to process might be considered more likely because a process has been put in place to reduce FTEs by changing job descriptions and requiring personnel reductions through attrition. Soft savings can move toward becoming hard if an effective benefits realization process is in place.

Task 7 is to filter the criteria.

"Of all the value calculations in a typical business case, experience shows that it is typically 3 or 4 (out of the 12) that ultimately drive the decision to invest or not. However, a dozen are needed so the decision team can pick and choose which ones they have the most confidence in" (Keen and Digrius 2003, 47). It is also important that criteria are included for each important group of decision makers. For example, the CFO and physician leaders may have different criteria and they need to be represented. However, having more criteria increases the work involved in preparing the business case and may blur the essential message about the value of the investment.

> "Of all the value calculations in a typical business case, experience shows that it is typically 3 or 4 (out of the 12) that ultimately drive the decision to invest or not" (Keen and Digrius 2003, 47). It is also important that criteria are included for each important group of decision makers.

Step Three: Align (Connect the Dots)

"Alignment is the process of keeping all activities and resources headed in the same direction in a mutually reinforcing manner" (Keen and Digrius 2003, 49). Senior management wants to know how strong the cause-and-effect relationship is between investing in an IT project and realizing key business objectives.

Task 8 is to align criteria.

"'Align criteria' is the process of first checking, then adjusting, for a compelling cause-and-effect relationship among successively higher-level decision criteria" (Keen and Digrius 2003, 50). For example, a criterion for making an investment in a medication administration check system that uses bar coding may be "to reduce the number of times a patient receives an incorrect medication." If another criterion (of great interest to the CFO) is "net revenue is increased because of shortened length of stay," the cause-and-effect relationship needs to be made clear. The fact that the hospital gains net revenues under prospective payment or capitation if length of stay is reduced needs to be highlighted.

Step Four: Calculate (Show the Money)

> **The key principles for this step are (Keen and Digrius 2003, 55):**
>
> - **Establish credibility with clear, believable calculations.**
> - **Explain every computation.**
> - **Cite convincing evidence for every assumption, reason, and conclusion.**
> - **Use agreed-upon estimates if no concrete data are available.**

Task 9 is to construct explanations, which include all text information concerning descriptions, evidence, references, and notes.

Task 10 is to define formula sets and variables.

Some mistakes include not providing exact formulas for calculating the savings presented, not defining the time period, and presenting a level of accuracy that is not believable (e.g., future savings of $248,897.69 instead of approximately $250,000).

Task 11 is to locate metrics and calculate them.

Sources of data include internal systems, other organizations that have implemented the technology, published literature, and expert judgment. Both the "Computerized Physician Order Entry at Brigham and Women's Hospital in Boston" and "Electronic Medical Records in Primary Care" studies described in chapter 1 provide examples of how each type of source can be utilized.

Step Five: Prove (Who Says So?)

"Proof is defined as evidence sufficient to convince someone that something is true or believable. Evidence is especially important in business cases because skepticism is high among people charged with approving IT investment requests" (Keen and Digrius 2003, 67).

Task 12 is to determine what types of proof are needed.

Keen and Digrius (2003, 70) present three primary elements in a line of reasoning:

1. Claims (assertions for which we wish to gain acceptance)
2. Grounds (evidence data to help prove our claims)
3. Warrants (reasons and shared values)

The proof for a claim that "reducing medication errors in the next six months is imperative" might be a recent Joint Commission inspection report or a statement from federal or state officials on their intention to conduct investigations. The proof for grounds such as "the number of adverse drug events has increased 20 percent in the last year" would be a recent internal study. The proof for a warrant such as "patient safety takes precedence over reducing budget deficits" might be a recent published affirmation of this presented at a board retreat.

Task 13 is to provide evidence from the sources identified in Task 11 that fits the needs identified in Task 12.

A large literature is available on the benefits of clinical applications (e.g., Shekelle, Morton, and Keeler 2006; MacDonald, Turisco, and Drazen 2003; U.S. Government Accountability Office 2003). Grounds that could be used to support development of decision support tools at an academic medical center could be Kaushal et al.'s (2006) example, mentioned earlier where they calculate savings related to renal dosing.

While this example appears to provide grounds for a claim that this intervention saves money, care still need to be taken to explain the logic being used; for example, why should we believe that these results would be achieved in our hospital?

Step Six: Analyze (Find the Winner)

"Analyze is the step where we discover what type of *information* has been created from all the data gathered—what recommendation should be made and why" (Keen and Digrius 2003, 74).

Task 14 is to review alignment and compute the final ROI.

This task deals with three activities (Keen and Digrius 2003, 75):

1. Realign: Recheck for a compelling cause-and-effect relationship between payoffs benefiting different levels of the organization.
2. Compute: Calculate the overall financial results, using IRR, NPV, ROI, and payback period (or whatever computations are requested by the decision team).
3. Compare: Match the financial results to the minimum acceptable standards (hurdle rates) for the enterprise.

Reviewing alignment requires a final check of the decision criteria alignment defined in task 8 to be sure that "each payoff area most effectively and logically supports one another" (Keen and Digrius 2003, 75). Taking the example of the medication administration check using bar coding described for task 8, here it is necessary to check that the logical cause-and-effect relationship between reduced medication errors and increased net revenue is clear and compelling. Has it been made clear what medication errors will be most affected and whether those errors are responsible for higher lengths of stay? Why would lower length of stay increase net revenue? Because patients who have an adverse drug event incur higher costs that are not reimbursed? Patients who are given the appropriate medication at the right time may also go home sooner. Are both effects being considered?

If the organization has set minimum financial results for investments, the results can now be compared to them. For example, a payback period of eighteen months or less and an ROI of at least 25 percent may be required.

Task 15 is to identify the key themes of the business case.

"A 'theme' is a dominant idea within a larger work. Themes are vital because they aid the audience in not only understanding but also accepting the messages in the subject matter. It is especially important to use themes in business cases when dealing with inherently risky IT investment options. Decision teams will never accept what they do not understand. The responsibility of the business case team is to discover key themes and communicate them to the decision team" (Keen and Digrius 2003, 81). A business case for providing wireless communication devices for nurses might have these themes:

- The devices will significantly shorten the time required for nurses, physicians, and other staff to locate each other and confer.
- Nurse and physician satisfaction will be significantly increased.

- Nurse retention could be positively affected, lowering overtime and agency nurse costs.
- Net revenue would increase because patient length of stay would be reduced as a result of improved work flow.

Keen and Digrius suggest that a business case should never have more than one major and two related, supporting themes. Looking at the example of wireless communication, the major theme could be improved communication and the two related themes could be lowered nursing costs and increased net revenue because of reduced patient LOS. The fact that nurse satisfaction would increase would be part of the justification for estimating higher nurse retention.

Task 16 is to determine recommendations.

The recommendations section of a business case (Keen and Digrius 2003, 85):

- Unequivocally specifies a recommendation
- Includes a time frame for the decision, that is, "immediately" (if that has emerged as an important issue in maximizing the value of the proposed investment)
- Summarizes major financially based tangible results known to be of high interest to the decision team
- Summarizes major intangible factors that reinforce the key value themes established for the business case
- Reflects the logical outcome of the analysis discussed in the business case
- Says it all in 50 words or less (so the decision team can cut to the chase)

Step Seven: Storytell (Explain It)

Step seven is to package the material "in a manner that accurately conveys the intended message of the business case and to do it in a way that is succinct and compelling" (Keen and Digrius 2003, 88). The key principles are to (Keen and Digrius 2003, 90):

- Convert key themes and data to visual media as much as possible.
- Build a logical sequence of topics.
- Speak the audience's language.
- Uncover and tell stories that illustrate key points.
- Encourage presentations and then prepare well with highly visual content.

Task 17 is to construct graphics and narratives consistent with the key principles.

Task 18 is to write "ROI stories."

"ROI storytelling is about relating people-oriented tales that illustrate a key theme, finding, or message of the business case" (Keen and Digrius 2003, 95). Good stories should match the audience and have one primary goal (Keen and Digrius 2003, 132). If the primary decision maker is a skeptical CFO, then the story might describe the efforts of the team to consult prominent experts to verify the assumptions used. The goal in this case would be to get buy-in from the CFO. If nurses are important to the success of the project, then a verbatim testimonial from a nurse at a hospital that has already implemented the technology could be the story, the primary goal of which would be to relieve anxiety or convince nurses that the added work would yield real benefits.

Task 19 is to define and give presentations.

It is important to focus on explaining the business case findings, not to try to sell the conclusions (Keen and Digrius 2003, 96).

> "At its core, the worth of a business case is not in its mass of numbers. A business case's value always springs from the quality of the guided conversation it stimulates about the shape of the future. Conversations move people to action. Data are merely the backdrop, although admittedly an essential one" (Keen and Digrius 2003, 91).

Resources

A searchable database of published studies of the cost and/or benefits of health information technology is available at http://healthit.ahrq.gov/tools/rand.

Finkler, Steven A. 2005. *Financial management for public, health, and not-for-profit organizations.* 2nd ed. Upper Saddle River, NJ: Pearson Prentice Hall.

Healthcare Financial Management Association and Cerner. 2005. EHR investments: The value case for senior healthcare financial executives. May. http://www.hfma.org/library/Information+Systems/Electronic+Health+Records/EHR_Investments400585.htm (accessed May 7, 2007). Offers advice on how to make a better business case for EHR adoption (see Exhibit 3).

References
for Chapters 1–3

Baldwin, Gary. 2000. CIO secrets to calculating return on investment. *Health Data Management* July: 55–67.

Bates, D.W., N. Spell, D.J. Cullen, et al. 1997. The costs of adverse drug events in hospitalized patients. *Journal of the American Medical Association* 277 (4): 307–11.

Benson, Robert, Thomas Bugnitz, and William Walton. 2004. *From business strategy to IT action.* Hoboken, NJ: John Wiley & Sons.

Boles, Keith, and Michael Cook. 2005. Investing in information technology. In *Strategic management of information systems in healthcare,* edited by Gordon Brown, Tamara Stone, and Timothy Patrick, 195–221. Chicago: Health Administration Press.

Briggs, Bill. 2006. Making the transition to filmless radiology. *Health Data Management,* November 20. http://www.healthdatamanagement. com/html/current/CurrentIssueStory.cfm?articleId=14215 (accessed November 29, 2006).

Classen, D.C., S.L. Pestotnik, R.S. Evans, et al. 1997. Adverse drug events in hospitalized patients. *Journal of the American Medical Association* 277 (4): 301–6.

Cusack, Caitlin, and Eric Poon. 2006. Evaluation Toolkit, Version 3. Point your browser to http://healthit.ahrq.gov/ and search for "Cusack Evaluation Toolkit" to access this source.

Dell Computer. 2006. Total cost of ownership. http://www.dell.com/ content/topics/global.aspx/tco/en/tco?c=us&cs=555&l=en&s=biz (accessed May 7, 2007).

Finkler, Steven A. 2005. *Financial management for public, health, and not-for-profit organizations.* 2nd ed. Upper Saddle River, NJ: Pearson Prentice Hall.

Frisse, Mark. 2006. Comments on return on investment (ROI) as it applies to clinical systems. *Journal of the American Medical Informatics Association* 13 (3): 365–67.

Healthcare Financial Management Association and Cerner. 2005. EHR investments: The value case for senior healthcare financial executives. May. http://www.hfma.org/library/Information+Systems/Electronic+Health+Records/EHR_Investments400585.htm (accessed May 7, 2007).

Jantos, Laura D. 2005. Analyzing the financial proposition: Developing a cost-benefit analysis. May. http://www.ecgmc.com/insights_ideas/pdfs/Developing_Cost-Benefit_Analysis.pdf (accessed November 8, 2006).

Kaushal, Rainu, Ashish Jha, Calvin Franz, et al. 2006. Return on investment for a computerized physician order entry system. *Journal of the American Medical Informatics Association* 13 (3): 261–66.

Keen, Jack, and Bonnie Digrius. 2003. *Making technology investments profitable: ROI road map to better business cases.* Hoboken, NJ: John Wiley & Sons.

Kian, Leslie, Michael Stewart, Catherine Bagby, and Jan Robertson. 1995. Justifying the cost of a computer-based patient record. *Healthcare Financial Management* 49 (7): 58–67.

MacDonald, Keith, Fran Turisco, and Erica Drazen. 2003. Advanced technologies to lower health care costs and improve quality. http://www.masstech.org/ehealth/reports.html (accessed November 9, 2006).

Mohr, David, and Jennifer Ferguson. 2005. Show me the benefits: Implementing an EHR. Paper presented at the Healthcare Information and Management Systems Society Annual Meeting, Dallas, TX, February 16, 2005.

Murphy, Tony. 2002. *Achieving business value from technology: A practical guide for today's executive.* Hoboken, NJ: John Wiley & Sons.

Schmitt, Karl, and David Wofford. 2002. Financial analysis projects clear returns from electronic medical records. *Healthcare Financial Management* 56 (1): 52–57.

Shekelle, P.G., S.C. Morton, and E.B. Keeler. 2006. Costs and benefits of health information technology. Technology Assessment No. 132, Agency for Healthcare Research and Quality Publication No. 06-E006. April. http://www.ahrq.gov/downloads/pub/evidence/pdf/hitsyscosts/hitsys.pdf (accessed November 1, 2006).

Sicotte, Claude, Guy Pare, Marie-Pierre Moreault, and Andre Paccioni. 2006. A risk assessment of two interorganizational clinical information systems. *Journal of the American Medical Informatics Association* 13 (5): 557–66. http://www.jamia.org/cgi/content/full/13/5/557 (accessed November 16, 2006).

Sublett, Patsy. 2005. The impact of bar code point-of-care medication administration on error reporting. Paper presented at the Healthcare Information and Management Systems Society Annual Meeting, Dallas, TX, February 15, 2005.

Swayne, Linda, W. Jack Duncan, and Peter Ginter. 2006. *Strategic management of health care organizations.* Malden, MA: Blackwell Publishing.

Taylor, Rick, John Manzo, and Mark Sinnett. 2002. Quantifying value for physician order-entry systems: A balance of cost and quality. *Healthcare Financial Management* 56 (7): 44–48.

U.S. Government Accountability Office. 2003. Information technology: Benefits realized for selected health care functions. October. http://www.gao.gov/cgi-bin/getrpt?GAO-04-224 (accessed November 9, 2006).

Wager, Karen, Frances Lee, and John Glaser. 2005. *Managing health care information systems: A practical approach for health care executives.* San Francisco: Jossey-Bass.

Wang, Samuel, Blackford Middleton, Lisa Prosser, et. al. 2003. A cost-benefit analysis of electronic medical records in primary care. *American Journal of Medicine* 114 (April 1): 397–403.

Case Study No. 2

NextCare Urgent Care: Implementing Computer-Based Patient Registration

NextCare Urgent Care (www.nextcare.com) operates twenty-seven immediate care clinics in Arizona, Colorado, North Carolina, and Georgia. In March 2005, Next-Care announced its decision to put kiosks in its clinics that would facilitate the patient check-in and triage process by allowing patients to enter information when they arrived. The kiosks were expected to result in higher patient satisfaction, improved patient throughput, and increased revenue because of improvements in billing. In 2007, NextCare plans to allow patients to enter the information online before coming to a clinic.

NextCare Urgent Care

NextCare Urgent Care was founded in 1993 by John Shufeldt, an emergency medicine physician who realized the need for an alternative to overcrowded emergency departments. NextCare's headquarters is in Mesa, Arizona.

NextCare's immediate care clinics treat non-life-threatening conditions such as cold, flu, allergies, sinus infections, earaches, eye infections, and minor burns or lacerations. Other services provided include drug screens; treatment for occupational injuries; physicals for school, sports, or employment; x-rays and other lab services; prescriptions filled on-site; and flu shots. Walk-ins are welcome seven days a week.

Patient Kiosks

NextCare began looking at electronic medical record products in 2002 and selected vendor NextGen (www.nextgen.com) because it had both EMR and electronic practice management (EPM) software that could enable exchange of information. An EPM takes care of the business operations, including billing, scheduling, and maintaining an appointment book. NextCare contracts with InforMed Medical Network to maintain and operate its NextGen EPM and EMR systems.

In March 2005, NextCare announced its decision to work with Galvanon (www.galvanon.com) to install kiosks to facilitate the patient check-in and triage processes. Galvanon was to supply all NextCare facilities with MediKiosk™ self-service systems (both hardware and software) to identify patients at check-in, gather necessary forms and signatures, and collect co-payments and outstanding balances. The kiosks would also be used to capture symptoms and medical histories, expediting the triage process and improving patient flow throughout the facility. An interface would automatically put information entered by patients into the clinic's EMR and EPM systems.

After six months, to obtain kiosk software more quickly, Next-Care asked InforMed and Simbiote Development (www.simbiote.com) to write a kiosk program in several phases. Phase one was to get a kiosk operating that would allow patients to enter information and for staff to receive and accept it. This phase is now live, and the information input through the kiosk system is automatically entered into the EMR. The screens for the kiosk program were based on information that was previously on paper forms (see figure CS2-1).

Patient Acceptance

Approximately 94 percent of patients use the kiosk. Of the 6 percent who do not use it, some patients do not feel they are well enough to enter the information themselves, and some elderly patients are resistant to using the kiosk.

Figure CS2-1. Data Entry Screen from NextCare Kiosk System

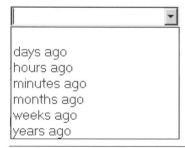

History of Present Illness
Please answer the questions below. Check all that apply to today's visit.

Is this a work related injury? ☐ Yes ☐ No

Select the primary reason for today's visit: [▾]

When did your symptoms begin: [⬍] [▾]   Did they begin: [▾]

Since your symptoms began, have they: [▾]

How often do you experience these symptoms: [▾]

How bad are your symptoms now: [▾]

Where are your symptoms located (check all that apply):

Side: [▾]

☐ Head	☐ Mouth	☐ Neck	☐ Wrist	☐ Abdomen/Stomach	☐ Knee	☐ Other
☐ Face	☐ Lips	☐ Shoulder	☐ Hand	☐ Pelvis/Bladder	☐ Leg	
☐ Eyes	☐ Gums	☐ Upper Arm	☐ Finger	☐ Genitals	☐ Ankle	
☐ Ears	☐ Tongue	☐ Elbow	☐ Chest	☐ Hip	☐ Foot	
☐ Nose	☐ Throat	☐ Lower Arm	☐ Back	☐ Thigh	☐ Toe	

Did they begin: (Pull-down menu)

[▾]
days ago
hours ago
minutes ago
months ago
weeks ago
years ago

Source: Reprinted with permission from NextCare Urgent Care.

Benefits

According to John Schufeldt, chief executive officer of Next-Care Urgent Care (2005), "By capturing this level of detail, our staff will be better prepared to identify which patients require immediate attention. This new approach to registration will also enable our facilities to reduce wait times for patients and improve overall operating efficiency."

Increased revenue could come from greater throughput per day. Improved documentation could result in changes in coding that increase revenue, allow bills to go out faster, and reduce denials. Some of the benefits are the result of both the kiosk system and the EMR and EPM systems that have been installed and interfaced. Harder-to-measure benefits would be increased volume because of greater customer satisfaction or the perception that NextCare provides superior service.

Increased Patient Throughput and Reduced Waiting

The kiosks relieve the bottleneck at the front desk. Provider downtime is reduced because patients move through the registration process faster. Patients sit at two to three kiosks near the front desk, allowing staff to work with several people at the same time. Staff no longer have to type in the information that patients write on paper forms. When patients did not answer questions or their handwriting could not be read, staff had to call patients back, leading to time lost that could otherwise be used helping patients. Typed information is more readable, and the software does not allow patients to continue unless they have completed all items. (See the sample error screens in figure CS2-2.) When patients return for a subsequent visit, they just have to verify or update the demographic and history information that appears on the kiosk screen.

The kiosks have increased the speed of the input process rather than reduced the number of staff needed. It took staff eight to ten minutes to enter all the patient data before the kiosk implementation. NextCare centers see approximately fifty patients per day, so the staff time saved is significant. Implementation of the kiosks has allowed staff to focus on other tasks, including increasing the number of insurance coverages they verify before the patient is seen, which helps cash collection (staff previously would let patients go to the exam room before verifying all coverages to keep the flow of patients moving). NextCare is now able to more accurately determine the patient's required co-payment and collect the deductible if it has not been satisfied.

Some patients leave before they are seen because they believe the wait is too long. Decreasing waiting times may result in a higher volume of patients and more revenue.

Figure CS2-2. Error Screens from NextCare Kiosk System

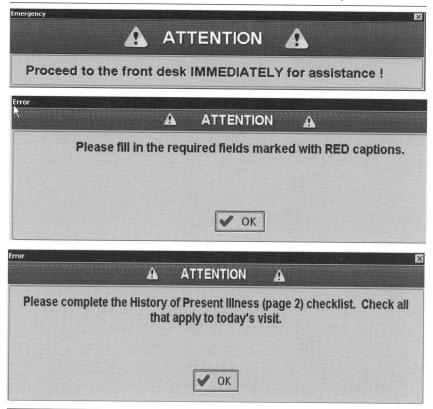

Source: Reprinted with permission from NextCare Urgent Care.

More Complete Documentation

The kiosks can improve documentation of the visit and the accuracy of the codes that determine payment. An interface with the EMR allows physicians to view information entered by patients at the kiosks. In a paper system, patients do not always complete questions, and office staff may still let them see the physician to keep the flow of patients moving. Similarly, physicians focus on patient care and sometimes skip a question that the patient has not answered. Documentation is now more complete because the kiosk software does not allow patients to move on without answering a question (see figure CS2-2). From a risk management perspective, the patients' own words are documented more frequently. What questions were asked and how the patient responded are made clear.

The patient will be asked for different information, based on gender or if the patient is a child. Questions for occupational medicine patients will be different if the visit is for an injury, a drug screening, or a pre-employment physical or if they say they are covered by worker's compensation.

Coding Accuracy and Justification

Financial benefits can be seen from having a more complete medical record. The accuracy of the codes that determine payment can be improved. Complete documentation to justify the code can speed up payment and avoid penalties after an audit.

Three components determine the level of service and, therefore, payment: history, exam, and medical decision. The physician considers these and assigns an evaluation and management code at the end of the visit. The codes represent five levels of acuity, evaluation, and management. These codes are reviewed by billing staff for appropriateness and may be reviewed by quality assurance (QA) staff to determine if the documentation is complete.

For the history component, the amount of information (e.g., social history, family history, past medical history) that the physician reviews can affect the code and, therefore, payment. For example, if the physician reviews information about the patient's smoking history and enters that in the chart, it can affect payment. They do not have to discuss it with the patient, they only have to review it. When the patient uses the kiosk, the physician does not have to type in the information, so it is more likely to be available. Codes may not be correct because information was not available, resulting in lost revenue if payment would have been higher. The kiosks help to get more complete information from the patient.

For example, documentation of a level four or five visit for a new patient requires a complete history, including the patient's social history, family history, and past medical care. Social history would include whether the patient had recently traveled abroad or had a history of smoking or alcohol use. Based on the patient's complaint, the physician would have to ask relevant questions. If the physician did not ask about social history, a level four or five code would not be justified, even if the exam was performed and the medical decision was correct.

Codes may also not be correct because there is no documentation that the information was reviewed. The EMR assists in improving coding and documentation by requiring that physicians click a box at the end of each section to signify that they have reviewed the information. In a paper system, physicians may also ask a question but not document the answer. In the EMR, the physician can more easily indicate the questions that were asked. Prompts appear to encourage them to answer. Typically, physicians use the computer as they are speaking with the patient. At a minimum, they review the information before seeing the patient.

A code may be correct, but there is insufficient documentation to justify it, resulting in a denial of payment or penalties if the records are audited. As described, both the kiosk system and EMR help to prevent that occurrence.

For example, the kiosk system allows NextCare to collect a complete history component before the visit. The information appears on the EMR when the physician opens it, and the physician has to affirm by checking a box that the patient's social history was reviewed before continuing. Unless they do that, reviewing the patient's social history would not affect the coding of the visit. If the physician does not check a box, he or she is redirected back to the appropriate page when trying to close out the chart.

In a paper chart, physicians were asked to sign the bottom of the page to indicate that they had reviewed the patient's social history. They did not always sign. Physicians would code the visit, but when charts were reviewed as part of QA, it would be determined that they had not signed the pages needed to justify the code. The EMR, therefore, also cuts down on the work required for QA. Staff at the front desk were asked to look through the chart to see if it was complete before discharging the patient, increasing patient wait times.

Payer Verification

Patients are not asked to type in insurance information at the kiosk because it takes a long time and they make mistakes, requiring staff to re-enter it. Rather, patients are asked for their insurance cards and photo identification, which are scanned. Staff then enter the required information.

Competitive Advantage

NextCare also wants to keep up with the competition in terms of customer service. Tracy Patterson, NextCare's executive vice president and chief development officer, says, "We want to be the best out there."

Cost

NextCare's contract with InforMed is based on a percentage of revenue. InforMed was willing to hire Galvanon and then Simbiote Development to write and implement the kiosk software at no additional charge because it agreed with NextCare that the system had the potential to increase revenue. The only additional costs to NextCare were for hardware and structural changes to the clinics. The kiosks themselves cost approximately $2,000 each (including touch-screen monitors, mice, keyboards, signature pads, and terminals with server connections). NextCare also paid for network installation costs, such as running Ethernet cables and adding wireless access points. There were also structural costs, including adding kiosk desks and reorganizing some lobbies, of approximately $500 per kiosk. Setup and configuration of the kiosks and the network was done by InforMed without any additional charge.

NextCare did not base the decision to proceed on the basis of cost, but the project was rolled out on a pilot basis to determine what the cost and return might be. The financial decisions for NextCare were:

- Which type of kiosk to select. Kiosks range in price from $2,000 to $15,000 each. Models include units at which people stand and mobile tablets (www.galvanon.com/products/medikiosk/hardware.htm).
- How quickly to implement kiosks at centers. The decision was partly based on estimates of kiosk cost and how quickly the costs would be returned if NextCare would be able to add one more patient per day.

The kiosks have been operating at the pilot site for one year. The centers in Arizona, Colorado, and Georgia are using them now, and the North Carolina centers are being converted. (Two of the NextCare centers are currently using the kiosks.)

Measuring Benefits

NextCare is starting to measure door-to-door time (time of check-in to time in the exam room to check-out time). The kiosk helps to accurately measure check-in time. The kiosk software records when the patient completed entering information and when it was accepted by staff. The EMR software records when the physician began reviewing the patient's information and when the patient was discharged. The information on patient waiting time can be compared to comment cards from patients, where waiting time is frequently a cause of dissatisfaction.

Door-to-door time and patient waiting time has, in general, gone down. Each clinic is given this information on a "scorecard" and is ranked against other clinics. Staff, including physicians, get bonuses based on rank. Because data are collected automatically by the kiosk, EMR, and EPM systems, the information cannot be falsified.

One difficulty has been separating the effects of the kiosks from other initiatives undertaken by NextCare. Those initiatives are designed to improve documentation and customer throughput. For example, it is difficult to separate the effect of the kiosk from the change stimulated by the scorecarding and ranking of clinics on door-to-door time.

NextCare has also changed the number of lab tests done on-site, adding complete blood count and the chemistry panel. Results are returned to the physician in under 15 minutes instead of the next day. Revenue from the tests themselves has, therefore, gone up.

Lab results can also change the code for the visit, as they can affect medical decision making. Insurers accept that if more tests were run to determine what was wrong with the patient, the medical decision-making component was more difficult. The complexity of the visits is determined by the number of diagnoses, which can increase based on lab results. Because physicians can see the results at the end of the visit, they can make a more appropriate choice on the level of difficulty of the visit. Lab tests to support coding are also more accurately documented in the record for that visit. If an increase in revenue has occurred due to coding changes, it is difficult to know what effect to attribute to the kiosks.

Staff time is saved because they no longer have to call patients to follow up on lab results. This has allowed staff to carry out other duties rather than reduced the number of staff.

The same difficulty in attributing changes to the kiosks exists for patient satisfaction. Patients may be more satisfied because of reduced waiting that results from other initiatives. But it may also be because their lab tests are available immediately, and they get a diagnosis in one visit instead of two.

Schufeldt believes the "ROI was obvious because the costs were relatively nominal and the upside in data collection, improvement in risk management and efficiency would be significant" (NextCare Urgent Care 2005).

Next Phase

The next phase of kiosk implementation will be to allow patients to enter the information online before coming to the urgent care center. This would expand the current Web check-in system, which now only asks for name, address, and employer information. The current Web check-in allowed NextCare to reroute patients to centers that were less busy, reducing wait times for patients. It also allowed NextCare to introduce new clinics into the market. Patients were still asked to come fifteen minutes earlier to fill out paperwork or use the kiosk, even if the paperwork took only five minutes.

When the new Web check-in process is fully implemented, patients will receive a phone call and be told what time to come and what room they will be seen in, so they are not waiting at a center but in the comfort of their home. Patients also will not have to wait next to someone with a contagious disease. They will not arrive and face a two-hour wait and perhaps leave.

The information collected may also indicate that the patient needs or wants a service outside the scope of the clinics—either low acuity (e.g., advice on how to prevent hair loss) or high acuity (e.g., a pacemaker adjustment)—or that the patient is insured by a noncontracted payer. For patient safety and to reduce liability, NextCare will always offer the patient the opportunity to come in and meet with a physician to discuss options. The submission of the information before arrival will allow for a phone call with a physician to discuss with the patient. It is assumed that many patients will decide not to come in, avoiding a nonbillable encounter.

Treating high-acuity patients who must be transferred to a hospital is a billable service, but reimbursement never pays the full costs involved, which include disruptions to the flow of patients in the clinic. Diverting those patients to emergency departments will, therefore, reduce costs.

NextCare expects that the improved Web check-in will reduce wait times and door-to-door times and also help increase the score, from good to excellent, on the customer satisfaction survey related to wait time.

In the future, information will also be collected online or at the kiosks in Spanish but appear in the EMR and EPM systems in both Spanish and English. Many questions require checking a box, making translation easier.

Bidirectional access to information is also in the future. In the beginning, patients will be able to enter information online but will not able to access information previously submitted to update it. Patients at the kiosks are currently able to do that.

Lessons Learned

Executive Vice President Patterson believes that organizations that want to implement a kiosk or online registration should:

- Measure scorecard components and door-to-door times before implementing the kiosk so that a baseline is established. Even a partial measurement or a few studies are helpful.
- Involve physicians from the beginning. Do not just involve IT staff.
- Remember that implementation will always take longer than expected.
- Talk to the IT department about what will be needed, such as memory and software upgrades.

Reference

NextCare Urgent Care. 2005. "NextCare Urgent Care Goes Self Service." March 7. http://www.nextcare.com/resource_center/press_selfserve.html (accessed May 7, 2007).

PART II

Project Management during Implementation

Introduction

THE CORNERSTONE tool for assessing and monitoring information technology (IT) projects is project management. It is an old adage that "you can't manage what you can't measure." Project management applies the appropriate measurement tools and then directs resources to manage their application on time and on budget. Without tight project management, projects are in constant jeopardy of missing their targets. We cannot emphasize this concept strongly enough. At the very beginning of any IT project, health care managers have to decide how formal their project management framework should be and what portion of the project budget needs to be allocated. Some health care organizations already require assignment of a trained project manager. Part III will help managers understand the benefits of incurring that cost.

A highly defined set of concepts and tools exist to manage the implementation of health care IT projects and to deal with the changes in scope, timeline, and budget that may be required. Managers need to also decide if any staff should be assigned to exclusively monitor projects and not participate in the work involved. They also need to decide if the organization should invest in "enterprise" project management software that allows anyone in the organization to see project information with just a Web browser and that permits the organized, even automatic, sharing of project information and tools for project management.

These decisions can only be made after the value of project management is assessed. Training, staff, and software require scarce dollars. This part of the book explores what project management tools exist and why they are considered important.

What All Hospitals Should Be Doing

- Hire a staff member certified in project management, or send someone for training.
- Create a project management office (PMO) even if it is staffed only by one person.
- The PMO should disseminate and provide education and consultation on a project management methodology.
- Discuss and agree on who can make decisions and who they must consult before money is spent on information technology. The chief executive officer (CEO) must lead this process.

Decisions

Health care managers must make a number of important decisions related to IT project management.

Should we create a PMO? A PMO should be in place that sets standards and monitors all projects. Given the size and growth of health care IT expenditures, the case for a PMO is persuasive and easy to make. Health care organizations need to define uniform project management practices and offer assistance to business units. Also obvious is the need to create accessible project status reports and an inventory of projects in order for the chief information officer (CIO) to maintain control.

What training is required? At least one member on any project team should be certified in project management or working on their certification. The Project Management Institute (www.pmi.org), for example, provides training toward project management professional (PMP) certification.

What control should the PMO have over projects? The need for a PMO that centralizes control of IT projects will depend on the organization's culture, the size and risk level of the IT projects being undertaken, and senior management's desire for a single point of accountability. At a minimum, the PMO should disseminate and provide education and consultation on a project management methodology. Services of a trained project manager (PM) should be offered to clinical and business units. Requiring the involvement of a trained PM is necessary to ensure that projects are completed on time and on budget.

How big should the PMO be? In smaller health care organizations the PMO may consist of one person and grow as responsibility is given to it. Regardless of the size and number of projects, it is oversight by someone, whose only responsibility is to monitor projects, that will make them successful.

Size is related to the role of the PMO. A "lite" or "repository" model PMO (which disseminates and provides education and consultation on a project management methodology) might be staffed by only a few people trained in project management methods, while a PMO that provides project managers will need to be larger.

In small organizations, the number and size of the IT projects each year may not justify even one full-time project manager. Such organizations should consider the benefits of project management for other types of projects not related to IT.

What return on investment (ROI) should we expect, and when? No evidence indicates that a PMO results in more projects that proceed on time and on budget in the first year. The rewards in that time frame are more likely to be an improved understanding of project status and resources consumed and a greater ability to prioritize projects. Benefits appear to improve over time. University Hospitals (UH) in Cleveland has seen an increase in the percentage of projects that are on time and on budget from 50 percent to 90 percent within three years (see the UH case study at the end of the introduction to this book). Implementation of changes in IT governance that accompany the creation of a PMO is a process that may lengthen the time for benefits to appear. Organizations may find that "coming up with a PMO that works for any given organization is an exercise in both customization and patience" (Santosus 2003).

Are changes in IT governance required? Who can make decisions and who must be consulted will need to change to achieve the benefits of a PMO. If project sponsors can continue to initiate projects without using the PMO, then the benefits of a PMO will not be gained. Using the PMO, however, will require changing the rules on when funds can be committed and spent. The benefits of using a trained PM will be lost if project sponsors can make decisions on changes in scope, timeline, and budget without consulting the PM. How one hospital system changed its IT governance is described in detail in the University Hospitals case study at the end of the introduction to this book.

4

What Is Project Management?

A HIGHLY DEFINED set of concepts and tools exists to manage the implementation of health care IT projects and to deal with the changes in scope, timeline, and budget that may be required. A number of textbooks specifically on information technology project management have been written (Schwalbe 2006; Richardson and Butler 2006; Garton 2004). Personal testimonies have also been published on information technology project management as an art (e.g., Berkun 2005). Yourdon (2004) has written on the challenges of IT projects with impossible time, money, and other constraints.

A study by the Standish Group (2001) describes the factors that most contribute to the success of information technology projects. In order of importance, they are:

- Executive support
- User involvement
- Experienced project manager
- Clear business objectives
- Minimized scope
- Standard software infrastructure
- Firm basic requirements
- Formal methodology
- Reliable estimates

Other criteria include small milestones, proper planning, competent staff, and ownership.

The University Hospitals (UH) case at the end of the introduction to this book demonstrates how many of these factors can come together to produce significant improvement in the percentage of projects that are completed on time and on budget. University Hospitals has changed its IT governance process to highlight executive support and to increase user involvement. University Hospitals has created a PMO that utilizes experienced project managers and project and portfolio management software. It requires formal scope and business plan documents that are prepared by project sponsors and trained project managers.

Certification in project management is offered by the Project Management Institute (www.pmi.org), which offers the PMP certification. Certification requires both professional experience and passing an exam. The Project+ certification offered by the Computer Technology Industry Association (CompTIA; www.comptia.org) requires passing an exam.

The Project Management Institute's (2004) *Guide to the Project Management Body of Knowledge (PMBOK)* defines nine knowledge areas in project management:

1. Scope management
2. Time management
3. Cost management
4. Quality management
5. Human resources management
6. Communications management
7. Procurement management
8. Risk management
9. Integration management

The first four knowledge sets are referred to as "core knowledge areas," while the next four are "facilitating knowledge areas." Integration management involves coordinating all of the other areas to ensure that all elements come together at the right times to complete a project successfully (Schwalbe 2006, 117).

Scope, time, and cost management are sometimes referred to as the "triple constraint" because the project manager must balance the three often-competing goals (Schwalbe 2006, 7).

We examine each and how project management methods assist in monitoring and controlling them. It could be argued that there is a "quadruple constraint" because quality also has to be controlled and monitored (Schwalbe 2006, 8). We assume that few project sponsors are willing to accept a reduction in quality, so the expectation is that scope, time, and budget will be adjusted to produce a high-quality result.

We also discuss communications management, because understanding what needs to be done will help managers decide what software tools are needed. We discuss later how "enterprise" software can help in communications in ways that stand-alone desktop software cannot. A longer discussion of all of the knowledge areas can be found in the books mentioned earlier. A summary of the tasks involved in quality, human resources, risk, and procurement management is in the appendix at the end of part II.

Scope Management

According to the Project Management Institute (2004, appendix F):

> Project Scope Management includes the processes required to ensure that the project includes all the work required, and only the work required, to complete the project successfully. Project Scope Management is primarily concerned with defining and controlling what is and is not included in the project. The Project Scope Management processes include:
> - Scope Planning—creating a project scope management plan that documents how the project scope will be defined, verified, and controlled, and how the work breakdown structure (WBS) will be created and defined
> - Scope Definition—developing a detailed project scope statement as the basis for future project decisions
> - Create WBS—subdividing the major project deliverables and project work into smaller, more manageable components
> - Scope Verification—formalizing acceptance of the completed project deliverables
> - Scope Control—controlling changes to the project scope

For an IT project, the project scope will include what software and hardware will be installed, the parts of the organization where the system will be available, what functions the system will perform, what tasks will be carried out by internal or vendor IT staff, and what tasks will be carried out by operations staff (e.g., managers and staff of a radiology unit). The purpose is to define what is to be done so a budget and timeline can be created and the responsibilities of the major parties defined. This is to address common problems when the scope is not defined, such as "IT will implement the system" and "we expected that it would do more than it really does." "Out of scope" activities may also be listed to prevent misunderstandings about what is being purchased (e.g., additional PCs are not included) or what functions are being performed (personal digital assistants are not supported).

A project scope document may be used to support initial approval or denial of the project and to help in prioritizing the project, and it is an important component of the project plan that is created after project approval. If a PMO is established, it will develop the scope management plan, create and disseminate templates for a scope document, and manage the process of controlling changes to the project scope. Change management is important to prevent *scope creep,* a gradual increase in project scope of which senior management is not aware and may not approve. This might include promising to make the system available to other parts of the hospital or adding functions to the software that result in additional vendor charges, internal labor costs, or additional hardware.

At University Hospitals (see the case study at the end of the book's introduction), the PMO develops a preliminary project scope that is used to decide whether to proceed. After a project is approved by a senior vice president, a more complete scope document or business plan is prepared (see figure CS1-1). The more detailed scope document is then used to create the project management plan on Clarity, the software product used to manage projects. Approved changes to project scope are stored on Clarity, where they can be viewed by project staff.

> Change management is important to prevent *scope creep,* a gradual increase in project scope of which senior management is not aware and may not approve.

Time Management

Project Management Institute (2004, appendix F) defines *project time management* as including:

> the processes required to accomplish timely completion of the project. The Project Time Management processes include:
> - Activity Definition—identifying the specific schedule activities that need to be performed to produce the various project deliverables
> - Activity Sequencing—identifying and documenting dependencies among schedule activities
> - Activity Resource Estimating—estimating the type and quantities of resources required to perform each schedule activity
> - Activity Duration Estimating—estimating the number of work periods that will be needed to complete individual schedule activities
> - Schedule Development—analyzing activity sequences, durations, resource requirements, and schedule constraints to create the project schedule
> - Schedule Control—controlling changes to the project schedule

Once the start and end dates for a project have been communicated, it is easy for anyone to determine if the project was implemented on time. Thus, on-time delivery has become a common metric for evaluating project success. To achieve on-time performance requires a series of steps, however, including the definition of what actually has to be done, an accurate estimate of the resources and time that will be required, and a process for controlling changes to the schedule.

Managers who are not technically trained have difficulty evaluating the accuracy of a project schedule. They need to rely on staff who have carried out similar projects to provide the information needed. However, managers can make sure that a process is in place for monitoring the schedule, for approving changes, and for learning from experience in previous projects. This is facilitated by a PMO and project management software.

> Project management software can produce and make accessible project schedules in graphical form. Even a manager with broad responsibilities can quickly determine if attention needs to be paid to the project.

Project management software can produce and make accessible project schedules in graphical form. Project dashboards can be produced that provide information on whether a project is on schedule using green (yes) or red (no) icons. Even a manager with broad responsibilities can quickly determine if attention needs to be paid to the project.

Figures CS1-2 and CS1-3 of the UH case are examples of project dashboards. To get more detail, project management software can produce Gantt charts that show when individual tasks are supposed to begin and end and which tasks are being carried out concurrently or are to follow each other. More complex network diagrams can be produced that show mandatory dependencies (what tasks must be completed before another can begin), discretionary dependencies (what tasks the project team would prefer to occur first), and external dependencies (activities outside of the project scope that must occur first).

One of the benefits of using an experienced manager and a PMO is that project sponsors do not have to examine this information and can simply view a project dashboard on a weekly or monthly basis. But this information is needed by the PM and is useful in explaining changes in the project schedule.

Learning from previous experience is an important part of time management. A project that took three months at one hospital might wind up taking five elsewhere. It is important for someone to understand why and to use that information in creating future project schedules. This research is more likely to be done and communicated to others when a PMO has been created. The PMO can act as a repository of knowledge that allows the creation of more realistic schedules or changes that improve performance.

Cost Management

> Project Cost Management includes the processes involved in planning, estimating, budgeting, and controlling costs so that the project can be completed within the approved budget. The Project Cost Management processes include:
> * Cost Estimating—developing an approximation of the costs of the resources needed to complete project activities
> * Cost Budgeting—aggregating the estimated costs of individual activities or work packages to establish a cost baseline
> * Cost Control—influencing the factors that create cost variances and controlling changes to the project budget. (Project Management Institute 2004, appendix F)

Anyone with access to the data can easily determine if a project was implemented on budget, so this is another common metric for determining the success of project management. Like time management, cost management consists of more that one task, and performance depends on accurately completing each of them. Having a common template and a process for ensuring that cost estimates are produced using a consistent methodology is important for the final result. A PMO and trained PMs can help ensure both consistency and accuracy in cost estimation and budgeting.

Cost estimation relies heavily on accurate information and experience. Many IT projects involve innovations with which managers have little experience. Relying solely on vendor estimates is problematic, as incentives exist to minimize some cost estimates (to make the sale) and overestimate others (when problems arise that are not covered in the contract). A PMO that collects historical data on previous projects can help produce more accurate estimates.

Managers should be aware that alternative methods of estimating the cost of IT projects are available. They should ask which method has been used, where the data came from, and what assumptions have been made. *Analogous* or *top-down estimates* use the costs of a previous project as the basis for an estimate. *Bottom-up estimates* or *activity-based costing* use the estimated cost of individual tasks. The sum of all the cost estimates is the total cost of the project. A detailed work breakdown structure is critical for an accurate estimate. A WBS is a list or diagram showing all tasks to be carried out in the project. *Parametric modeling* uses selected project characteristics—for example, lines of programming code—to determine project costs. An estimate of $50 per line of code and the expected number of lines could be used to estimate total project costs, for example (Schwalbe 2006, 259–60).

Reserves, also called *contingency allowances,* will be shown as costs in many cost estimates. Their inclusion, however, may cause the estimate to be too high. "Contingency reserves are estimated costs to be used at the discretion of the project manager to deal with anticipated, but not certain, events. These events are 'known unknowns' and are part of the project scope and cost baselines" (Project Management Institute 2004, section 7.1.3). These reserves also need to be monitored and adjusted. For example, when the event for which the contingency was budgeted has passed, the reserves can be reduced.

A PM can serve as budget monitor and source of accurate information. While the finance department will be aware of the approved budget and invoices as they are received, the PM is also aware of approved changes in project scope and timeline that are needed to understand the financial condition of the project. For example, if a hardware vendor communicates that shipment will be delayed, the PM can estimate what that will do to the budget for the project. The change may mean incurring additional costs for consultants because project staff will have to be working on other projects until the hardware arrives. The PM can also work to determine if the shipment can be received more quickly and if the contract with the vendor allows for compensation for delayed shipment. This is one example of how the PM can assist in cost control.

> Time, scope, and cost management are interdependent. A project with a poorly defined scope (or where inappropriate scope creep occurs) will result in unexpected cost increases. Likewise, failure to create an accurate timeline will result in cost increases. A trained PM who accurately estimates and monitors time and scope can control costs.

Communications Management

As the Project Management Institute (2004, appendix F) defines it:

Project Communications Management includes the processes required to ensure timely and appropriate generation, collection, distribution, storage, retrieval, and ultimate disposition of project information. The Project Communications Management processes provide the critical links among people and information that are necessary for successful communications. Project managers can spend an inordinate amount of time communicating with the project team, stakeholders, customer, and sponsor. Everyone involved in the project should understand how communications affect the project as a whole. Project Communications Management processes include:
- Communications Planning—determining the information and communications needs of the project stakeholders
- Information Distribution—making needed information available to project stakeholders in a timely manner
- Performance Reporting—collecting and distributing performance information, including status reporting, progress measurement, and forecasting
- Manage Stakeholders—managing communications to satisfy the requirements of, and resolve issues with, project stakeholders

The Standish Group (2001), as mentioned earlier, identifies the top two factors related to project success as executive support and user involvement. Effective communications is essential for achieving both, and the content and the method of communications are important to the process. Stakeholders need to get the information they want and need in a way that suits their preferences. The IT world is rife with jargon, but that should not be an obstacle that leads to the attitude, "IT will take care of it." Nor should those involved in the project be inundated with detailed paper reports they neither want nor need.

As described in the UH case study, the organization decided that a monthly dashboard (figure CS1-2) should be sent by e-mail as a PDF file to a large group, while weekly dashboards for individual projects should be provided to project sponsors (figure CS1-3). The dashboards use colors to signal whether expectations in regard to the timeline and budget are being met. Staff working on the project can also access information by logging on to Clarity, the project management software. Project managers use e-mail to inform project sponsors and those working on the project when issues arise and alert them to the need for telephone calls and face-to-face meetings. University Hospitals has, thus, made decisions about each of the four processes identified by the Project Management Institute listed above, demonstrating that it is important that formal decisions be made on each process—for example, who will get what information when.

Communications management is an important component in selecting software to support project management. (The selection of such software is discussed in detail later.) Some important questions to be asked are detailed below.

Which stakeholders will be accessing information using the software? If the expectation is that anyone involved in the project can access information, reports must be easy to retrieve or produce. What the user sees should depend on what their role is in the process, both to simplify retrieval and to ensure they see only the appropriate information. To avoid miscommunication, only one database of information should exist. These requirements will mean purchasing enterprise software that is available over a network or via the Internet. If just a few project managers will be using the software to produce reports, less expensive desktop software may be sufficient.

Is the software going to be the primary method of communication among team members? Some organizations may prefer to use their existing e-mail system for communications and to store documents on an existing intranet. Others may want the software to serve as a virtual office for team members, who will use it for the majority of their communication. If the latter is true, then enterprise project management software is needed rather than less expensive desktop software used by individuals on their own computers.

It is possible to communicate about a project using e-mail and placing documents in a location accessible to those involved, for example, a shared hard drive. Team members and project sponsors may also prefer telephone calls and face-to-face meetings. Less expensive desktop project management software may suffice so that project managers can store information and produce reports.

Project Integration Management

The Project Management Institute (2004, appendix F) states:

> Project Integration Management includes the processes and activities needed to identify, define, combine, unify and coordinate the various processes and project management activities within the Project Management Process Groups. In the project management context, integration includes characteristics of unification, consolidation, articulation and integrative actions that are crucial to project completion, successfully meeting customer and stakeholder requirements and managing expectations. The Project Integration Management processes include:
> - Develop Project Charter—developing the project charter that formally authorizes a project
> - Develop Preliminary Project Scope Statement—developing the preliminary project scope statement that provides a high-level scope narrative

- Develop Project Management Plan—documenting the actions necessary to define, prepare, integrate, and coordinate all subsidiary plans into a project management plan
- Direct and Manage Project Execution—executing the work defined in the project management plan to achieve the project's requirements defined in the project scope statement
- Monitor and Control Project Work—monitoring and controlling the processes required to initiate, plan, execute, and close a project to meet the performance objectives defined in the project management plan
- Integrated Change Control—reviewing all change requests, approving changes, and controlling changes to the deliverables and organizational process assets
- Close Project—finalizing all activities across all of the Project Process Groups to formally close the project

In one sense, project integration management is carrying out a series of tasks that create, execute, and end a project. For example, writing a brief project charter formalizes the process of creating a project and establishes who will be accountable for it. In another sense, integration management is the coordination of all of the activities in the project that we have just discussed, for example, time and scope management.

> **The central assumption is that one individual—the project manager—is necessary to ensure that project integration occurs. To ensure that this process is carried out completely and consistently, that person needs to be trained in project management.**

In the next chapter, we define a unit in the organization that is responsible and accountable for project management.

5

Project Management Offices

PROJECT MANAGEMENT offices are units within an organization dedicated to the management of projects. The PMO can be composed of internal staff, staff from an outsourcing firm, or vendor staff.

Project Management Office Models

Gartner Research has defined a continuum of styles that range from a "lite" or "repository model," which collects and disseminates project management methodology and best practices, to a "strong manager" or "enterprise" model, which provides project managers to run projects. In an intermediate "coach" model, the PMO acts as trainer, consultant, or mentor, but project performance is actively monitored (Light et al. 2005, 9). Regardless of the model, "the first objective of a project office is the establishment of standard practices for measuring project performance and the development of a capability for understanding the status of key initiatives" (Light et al. 2005, 10).

Project management offices can develop and disseminate a consistent and standardized project management methodology, and they can select and maintain project management software tools. As an alternative to either waiting to be asked for help or taking control, the PMO can make available elements of the methodology (e.g., a template for project scheduling) to anyone while making project status reports accessible throughout the organization. The PMO can also collect information on the portfolio of IT resources and projects in the organization, helping senior management to prioritize projects. A risk in developing a PMO that only monitors projects, and does not work on them, is hostility within the organization as late, overbudget, or nonperforming projects are identified. This result could prevent the PMO from moving into a supportive role.

Some organizations may not want to create a PMO because it adds a unit to an already complex organization. They may also feel that PMO project managers will not become effective team members because they report to a PMO director and work on multiple projects. The challenge those organizations will face is how to perform the functions of a PMO without creating one. These functions include developing, disseminating, and ensuring compliance with a project management methodology; effectively applying project management software tools; and collecting and reporting accurate, timely, and comparable data on projects. We recommend that hospitals create a PMO, even if that means starting with one person and a "lite" or repository model.

Defining a Project

The organization needs to decide what constitutes a *project*. In the University of Illinois case described later in this chapter, a project was defined as work requiring 40 hours or more of staff time. Requests that would require less time could be accepted or rejected by IT directors without review by the IT council or PMO.

University Hospitals in Cleveland defines a project based on three basic criteria:

1. Whether or not it has strategic importance to UH
2. Whether or not it represents a capital expense
3. Whether or not it will require more than 90 calendar days and more than 120 Information Technology and Solutions department hours of effort to complete

Strategic importance is defined as (1) affecting multiple entities, (2) a change in technology, (3) a replacement of system(s), or (4) containing measurable/sustainable ROI. Projects that fail to meet any of the three basic criteria are defined as "service requests" and are sent to the appropriate applications manager.

University Hospitals's intent is to limit the number of projects that must move through its governance process, which is described in detail in the case study at the end of the introduction to this book. That process potentially slows down the implementation of the project. By setting the resource threshold at 40 or more hours of staff time, the University of Illinois Medical Center not only increases the work of the PMO but also increases control over staff resources. Defining a project is an important issue related to the degree of control that management wants over the project and resources as well as to determining the resources that must be allocated to the PMO.

Information Technology Governance

Information technology governance is a complicated subject that goes beyond the scope of this book (Weill and Ross 2004). We assume that a governance structure for IT exists that includes an IT council composed of the CIO and senior managers from finance, nursing, and operations. Project and portfolio management (PPM) is not governance, and PMOs are not the governing body for IT.

> "IT governance" specifies the decision-making authority and accountability to encourage desirable behaviors in the use of IT. IT governance provides a framework in which the decisions made about IT issues are aligned with the overall business strategy and culture of the enterprise. Governance is about decision making per se—not about how the actions resulting from decisions are executed. Governance is concerned with setting directions, establishing standards and principles, and prioritizing investments; management is concerned with execution. Thus, IT governance is a framework for decision making. It does not involve the underlying actions or processes that may result from the actual decisions made using the framework. It sets direction but does not direct the management of actions and processes related to executing on the decisions. (Stang 2006a, 7)

The PMO is, therefore, never a decision-making body in regard to project approval and setting or changing budgets or staff allocation. The primary role of the PMO in relation to the IT council is to assemble and report data and to provide analyses that help the council make decisions. The PMO can be called on to make recommendations. It can also help to enforce decisions made by the council in regard to budgets by reporting actual expenditures in relation to the budget.

However, as noted earlier, who can make decisions and who must be consulted will need to change to get the benefits of a PMO. If project sponsors can continue to initiate projects without using the PMO, then the benefits of a PMO will not be achieved. But requiring the use of the PMO will have to be enforced. One way is to change the rules on when funds can be committed and spent. University Hospitals has mandated that the only way to access funds from the capital budget is to send a proposal through the governance process. If it meets the definition of a project, then it is managed by the PMO or, for very large projects, a single dedicated project manager on the UH staff.

The benefits of using a trained project manager will also be lost if project sponsors can make changes in scope, timeline, and budget without consulting the PM. Governance concerns not only how projects are initiated but also how they are managed during implementation. Requiring project sponsors who own the funds to consult with anyone else may represent a significant change in the culture of an organization.

So while the PMO is not a decision maker, changes in the governance process that define how decisions are made are critically important for receiving the benefits of having a PMO.

> **Who can make decisions and who must be consulted will need to change to get the benefits of a PMO. If project sponsors can continue to initiate projects without using the PMO, then the benefits of a PMO will not be achieved.**

Strategic Alignment

Much has been written on the importance of ensuring that information technology supports the strategy of organizations. This is considered essential not only for reaping the benefits of investment in IT but also for ensuring that IT gets the support of senior management and boards of directors. A PMO can play a supporting role by maintaining data that allow investments to be categorized according to the strategy they support. It can help senior management answer questions such as, "What IT investments were made that support improvements in patient safety?" The PMO is not, however, usually a source of ideas on how to leverage technology to achieve strategic objectives. This is the job of managers, often assisted by outside consultants.

Portfolio Management

The collection of data on current and planned projects (e.g., budgets, start and end dates) just described is part of a process called *portfolio management* and is a distinct function or "module" of enterprise PPM software.

Portfolio management involves seven essential activities (Pickens and Solak 2005, 21):

1. Opportunity identification
2. ROI forecasting and value definition
3. Project prioritization
4. Capacity planning
5. Work scheduling
6. Program and project management and execution
7. Project performance and value assessment

These activities require the collection of data on all current and planned projects. Project and portfolio management software allows managers to create multiple scenarios that show the effect of possible changes in the portfolio of projects. For example, the CIO may want to know what effect the phased implementation of an electronic health record would have on staffing needs given the current set of active projects. Such an analysis might point out the need for adding database administrators or changing the start dates of projects. Project and portfolio management software permits managers to view in graphical form the impact of adding and deleting projects or changing start and end dates.

As noted earlier, PPM software can also be used to track the number of projects related to individual organizational strategies. Judgments about complexity and risk can also be added to allow managers to assess the entire portfolio on these variables. Project and portfolio management software allows managers to answer such questions as, "Over time, has the number of more complex and risky projects increased, which may result in an increasing number of projects whose timeline, scope, and budget will need to be adjusted?" If the answer is yes, then it may explain the number of changes that are occurring rather than signaling a failure in the project management process.

Developing the capability to support portfolio management can be the initial task of a PMO or the goal to which the PMO aspires. The argument for the former is that it assists senior management and boards of directors in making resource allocation decisions. As noted earlier, this role can increase resistance or decrease support for a PMO that starts out by enumerating delayed, overbudget projects without offering support. Organizations may instead choose to initially focus on implementing project management and moving to portfolio management as the PMO matures. Portfolio management will, therefore, serve to present a holistic view of an increasing number of successful projects while offering improved tools for making decisions on the priority of new projects.

Value of Project Management

No studies of PMOs have been undertaken in health care organizations. An online survey was conducted in 2003 by *CIO Maga-*

zine and the Project Management Institute (PMI), in which CIOs, chief technology officers, vice presidents in charge of IT, and PMI members were invited to take part, resulting in 303 responses from companies operating a PMO. Half of the respondents said the PMO had improved project success rates. The length of time that the PMO had been operating was related to project success rates. Respondents with PMOs in operation for more than four years reported a 65 percent success rate increase (Santosus 2003).

> **When asked about the top benefits of having a PMO, survey respondents listed implementation of project management standards (62 percent), increased internal customer satisfaction (38 percent), increased employee productivity (39 percent), lower costs (27 percent), and increased external customer satisfaction (25 percent) (Ware 2003).**

Metrics that companies have used to measure the effectiveness of a PMO include the accuracy of cost estimates, accuracy of schedule estimates, and project stakeholder satisfaction. Cancellation, postponement, and the scaling back of small projects are other measures. Giving the CIO the status and financial details of all IT projects could also be viewed as a measure of success (Santosus 2003). A PMO that wants to improve project manager skills needs a systems that measures skills.

While the University of Illinois Medical Center did not report an increase in the number of projects that were on time and on budget one year after creating a PMO (Isola, Polikaitis, and Laureto 2006), University Hospitals reported an increase from 50 percent to 90 percent in three years. This is consistent with the *CIO Magazine*/PMI survey in which respondents reported that the length of time that the PMO had been operating was related to project success rates (Santosus 2003).

Another measure of the value of a PMO is the extent to which IT staff and clinical and business staff are freed to do their jobs instead of performing project management tasks they were never trained to do. This is a difficult benefit to measure, as activity and cost accounting systems do not often break out project management as a distinct activity. Increased productivity would need to be assessed to detect the impact of the PMO.

In our experience, the cost of a PMO will range from 5 to 10 percent of a $10 million capital budget dedicated to projects. While the PMO may first be viewed as an additional cost, it should be remembered that money is already being spent on project management but not identified as such. Because trained project managers are more efficient, the cost of project management may actually be decreasing while the productivity of staff, relieved of project management tasks, may be increasing.

Because the PMO applies a consistent methodology across all projects, the extent to which projects are completed on time and on budget and the reasons for any changes can be determined. Without a PMO, data collection and project monitoring are likely to be inconsistent, making it difficult for senior management to monitor projects and understand the reasons for failure to meet expectations.

Finally, organizations need to consider whether project management is resulting in projects that are more successful in delivering their intended benefits, and not just on time and on budget. The CEO of University Hospitals noted that he would not build a building without an architect and an engineer; likewise, he would not undertake a major project without a project manager. The assumption is the same, which is that a trained professional produces a better project.

In the end, hard data on PMO benefits are not available. Project management offices are likely to appeal to organizations that have experienced significant project failures, but PMOs should be considered an important way to improve operations by all organizations.

Effective Practices

When asked which project management practices were most effective in helping the organization meet its financial goals, respondents to the *CIO Magazine*/PMI survey most frequently answered providing standard methodology for managing projects (56 percent), having responsibility for process and project reporting and tracking (38 percent), ensuring that similar projects are executed in a similar way (37 percent), having the funding and information needed to speed up or slow down project delivery (29 percent), and providing a process for resource allocation and capacity management (27 percent) (Ware 2003).

When asked about the most effective practices for helping the company meet its strategic goals, survey respondents listed, in this order, ensuring PMO projects have direct links to the company's strategic and operating plans (43 percent); providing standard methodology for managing projects (40 percent); having executive sponsorship/support from senior management (37 percent); ensuring that the PMO works only on projects that support a business goal or strategy (37 percent); and using a process to ensure that groups are aligned on project process, selection, priority, and execution (31 percent) (Ware 2003).

When asked to rank the top challenges to their PMO's effectiveness, *CIO Magazine*/PMI survey respondents listed, in this order, unreasonable workloads (52 percent), a lack of PMO authority to carry out objectives (43 percent), and a lack of support from business unit management (42 percent) (Ware 2003). These problems could be the result of inadequate specification of the role of the PMO. Gartner Research indicates that a PMO needs a charter that defines what it will or will not do, who it reports to, and what functions it will perform (Light et al. 2005, 13).

Responsibilities and Accountability

The degree of control that the PMO should have over project resources and schedules is an important decision. An enterprise or "strong manager" PMO, with project managers in charge of projects, may result in significant and damaging resistance from IT and other staff. On the other hand, such a PMO can be used by senior management to better control the use of resources and improve project success rates.

Meyer (2005) argues that "the proper role of a PMO is to help everybody become a good project manager—not to be a project manager for a few big projects." Its role is to "empower others with advice, training, methods, tools and services that make everybody successful at delivering their projects." Meyer believes that PMOs that try to manage projects are ultimately forced to manage only a few big projects for lack of resources, leaving smaller projects adrift. The PMO project manager becomes the controller of other people's resources, disempowering them and creating resentment. Creative ideas are lost, and staff become demoralized. Project management office PMs may also not be technically competent to make decisions but end up making the final judgments. This may result in "solutions that may have been delivered on time and on budget, but did not fit the technical architecture, were not in keeping with other managers' technology strategies and were difficult to support" (Meyer 2005).

> Meyer (2005) argues that "the proper role of a PMO is to help everybody become a good project manager—not to be a project manager for a few big projects."

Meyer sees the PMO as a "subcontractor" to the real project manager in the appropriate business unit. The PMO can help in this capacity at two levels. First, it can help others plan the steps in the process (e.g., by providing Gantt charts) and how they will control project resources. This can be just at the beginning or throughout the project. Second, it can help others administer project-specific data, reporting project status in a consistent way. Rather than the PMO serving as the controller, the CIO contracts internally and holds each subcontractor accountable for the delivery of components (Meyer 2005).

Meyer is clearly rejecting the strong manager model, but the coach model fits his description. However, to get the information needed to manage multiple projects, the PMO needs to be more than a coach and consultant. Standardized processes for measuring performance and results have to be established and enforced. Rather than defining how resources will be allocated, for example, the PMO can define when, how, and where resource use will be reported using a standard software product. The PMO can train staff in those processes. It can also operationalize the concept of portfolio management by compiling an inventory of IT resources and selecting and maintaining the tools needed to compare proposed projects in terms of their contribution to fulfilling the strategies of the organization. The information and analysis compiled by the PMO can be used to resolve resource conflicts and coordinate projects that depend on each other. "A good PMO can also provide organizational learning about why projects crash, and thereby prevent future difficulties" (Light et al. 2005, 6).

The PMO created by UH and described in the case study at the end of the introduction to this book fits neither the strong manager model nor the coach model. It also does not fit the repository or lite model described earlier. The PM at UH is accountable for the process, but not solely responsible for the work. The CEO and CIO of UH want the project sponsor to be "singularly accountable" for the project. But the project sponsor expects the PM to do most of the work of managing the project. However, PMs rely on project sponsors to "acquire" staff resources for the project, which means supporting the PM in requests for IT staff and ensuring that their own staffs are available. Each party in the process has penalties and rewards, which are expected to lead them to perform. University Hospitals has outsourced the PMO to First Consulting Group (FCG), and FCG pays a financial penalty if projects experience changes in budget and if "go live" dates have not been approved. The key element is a formalized governance process with strong executive support.

Defining the role of the PMO is, therefore, an important decision that needs to be based on the resources, goals, and culture of the organization. How a PMO is organized and staffed depends on "myriad . . . organizational factors, including targeted goals, traditional strengths and cultural imperatives" (Santosus 2003). For example, an organization whose culture stresses the autonomy of business units may wish to adopt a consultative model, while another organization faced with a complex, expensive, high-risk implementation (a new electronic health record or replacement of a financial system) might adopt a more centralized approach.

Regardless of the model selected, it is important for everyone to understand what the PM does. This should be made clear in the project scope document and later in the project plan. Berkun (2005) recommends a conversation between the PM and every member of the team in which three lists are made, enumerating what the PM does, what they both do, and what the team member does.

"In fact," writes Scott Berkun in *The Art of Project Management,* "in most cases, there is great ignorance among the technical folks about what the PM is doing all day, and without some kind of role discussion, they have no way of ever discovering what the PM is doing (and because PMs often do a lot of work to protect programmers and testers from politics, bureaucracy, and general management stupidity), the rest of the team might never have the opportunity to understand how much the PM is helping" (Berkun 2005, 179).

At UH, the project scope document defines the roles of the project sponsor, the PM, and team members in specific terms (see the UH case study, figure CS1-1).

Implementation of a Project Management Office at the University of Illinois Medical Center

The University of Illinois Medical Center established a PMO in 2004. The new CIO had been told by the CEO that the information systems (IS) department "never hits the dates they set . . . causes more problems after an upgrade than they fix . . . appears to be an add on cost . . . does not drive financial benefits with technology improvements" (Isola, Polikaitis, and

Laureto 2006). The relationship between IS and the business units was, "IS decided, IS took the lead, IS forced it, and IS took the blame" (Isola, Polikaitis, and Laureto 2006, 80).

The CIO believed a PMO was needed because "I could not value the number of requests that we were doing, we did not have an agreement on scope once we started a project, there was no formal governance structure, no project request process, nor any project prioritization process. In addition, we have a great IS team . . . that just did not know how to say 'we really can't do that . . . right now'" (Isola, Polikaitis, and Laureto 2006, 81). The fiscal 2006 IS plan identified 131 unprioritized projects. Most had no budgets, and none had ROI calculations.

A PMO was established with two dedicated full-time equivalent staff who were sent to a three-day course on project management. The PMO "was to manage IT projects as a portfolio of business investments; develop IT strategic plans; centralize management and coordination of projects and resources; formalize the project proposal and prioritization process; standardize project methodology and tools; and establish metrics on how IT investments are performing" (Isola, Polikaitis, and Laureto 2006, 82).

The PMO, therefore, fits the model of a centralized organization assisting senior management in the development and implementation of IT strategy while also setting and attempting to change project management standards. For example, a Web form was created on the intranet for submitting new IS requests. Requests that require more than 40 hours to complete (the definition of a project) are submitted to a project management council, which includes all IS staff leading projects and the CIO. A "phase zero" was introduced that requires estimates of scope, resources needed, costs, potential benefits, and risks. End dates or go-live dates are released only after phase zero is complete (Isola, Polikaitis, and Laureto 2006, 83).

However, the goal was for departments to take ownership and work collaboratively with the IS department. An IS advisory group with executives from operational areas (e.g., nursing, radiology) reviews information from phase zero to help set priorities. Project management office staff are not direct managers of projects who can over-rule project staff.

The results cited after one year were the development of a strategic plan, collaborative relationships between IS and medical center managers, and greater customer satisfaction because medical center managers believed that their input was sought. Medical center leadership now had a way to view the entire portfolio of IT investments and to quantify IT activities (Isola, Polikaitis, and Laureto 2006, 84)

The PMO has been less successful in other areas. Nearly every new request is absorbed by the IT department so that staff are overcommitted and projects are delayed. Benefit estimates are rarely available and, therefore, not considered. The PMO has "had only a modest effect on project management processes" (Isola, Polikaitis, and Laureto 2006, 85). Plans for year two included the implementation of a project management tool to automate components of the project management methodology. More training in project management was planned to expose all staff to the methodology.

The University of Illinois Medical Center appears to have avoided the problems raised by Meyer (2005) by not making the PMO responsible for actual project management. On the other hand, creation of the PMO has not, at least in the first year, resulted in a demonstrated improvement in the number of projects completed on time. Yet important problems have been addressed, including the absence of information on which to base decisions and a lack of involvement by managers outside of IT in project prioritization. The University of Illinois's experience in the first year appears to confirm Santosus's (2003) contention that "PMOs won't give organizations a quick fix or deliver immediate, quantifiable savings."

It may also be true that a more centralized model in which the PMO controlled projects would have delivered better results. This would have required a significant change in how work was done and recognition of the risks discussed by Meyer (2005) of lower performance by IT project staff. A centralized PMO would also have to have more staff, either transferred or new.

The CIO gave the two-person PMO work on the IT strategic plan, which must have consumed much of their time in the first year. It would be reasonable to expect that PMO staff would not be able to develop, disseminate, and advocate for significant change in how projects were managed.

6

Project and Portfolio Management Software

ROJECT AND PORTFOLIO management software is available to support the tasks involved in the nine areas described earlier in the Project Management Institute's *PMBOK*. This includes the three core functions of time management, resource management, and cost management. For example, such software can assist in time management by storing and allowing easy maintenance of a project timeline; requests for and approval of changes can be stored; and the software can support communications management by storing documents related to the project.

> **PPM software supports the PMO and makes it successful.**

A major difference between individual desktop software and enterprise products is the degree to which they support communication by allowing multiple people to use and maintain the same information, for example, a project budget. Products also differ in the extent to which they contain or provide links to e-mail, instant messaging (chat), and bulletin boards.

More complex (and expensive) software supports portfolio management by providing a single view in graphical form of all active and planned projects. As discussed earlier, this feature can assist managers in understanding how resources are being allocated to address each organizational strategy and allow for simulation of the effect of changing project start and end dates. Judgments about risk can be entered that can assist senior management and boards of directors to adjust the portfolio, much as an individual or bank would adjust a financial portfolio to fit their risk tolerance.

What Is Available

Products range from single desktop systems (e.g., Microsoft Project Standard) to enterprise software that allows users throughout an organization to retrieve and submit information and create and review reports. Microsoft Project is available in an enterprise version (Microsoft Enterprise Project Management Solution), and many other programs are available, including Computer Associates's Clarity (www.niku.com), Mercury Project and Portfolio Management Center (www.mercury.com), and Primavera (www.primavera.com). Enterprise products are installed on the organization's computers and require the operation of a server and database management software. Vendors also offer access to their products over the Internet (e.g., eProject; www.eproject. com), allowing organizations a lower initial cost and the opportunity to add modules as needed without further hardware costs.

Some PPM software generates a dashboard, which shows the current status of one or more elements of a project or group of projects. Figures CS1-2 and CS1-3 in the UH case study present dashboards for all projects and for a single project. Dashboards may reduce the time necessary for monitoring projects, as they present a few agreed-upon measures believed to be associated either with desired performance or with identifying risks requiring management attention. Some PPM software allows the manager to drill down—that is, click on the metric and immediately see the variables that are used to calculate it or are related to it. If this function is not available, the manager needs to view or create other reports or search a database for the desired information.

Access to information, including dashboards, can be *role based,* which means that individuals can access different information because of the role they have in the project. A programmer working on the project might be able to see the timeline and issues, but not the budget, for example. Project managers might be able to view the projects they are working on, while only the

PMO director and senior management can access information on all projects.

Communication of reports and dashboards can be either automatic or on demand, and it may be done by using the PPM software or external e-mail. At UH, project managers disseminate weekly a PDF file of the dashboard for individual projects to those overseeing or working on each project via Microsoft Outlook (figure CS1-3). Each month the CIO disseminates via e-mail a PDF of a dashboard showing all projects to a wide range of managers inside and outside of the IT department (figure CS1-2). Both UH managers and staff at the PMO can also log on to the Clarity PPM application and view dashboards, but which ones they can access will depend on their role.

Selecting Project and Portfolio Management Software

> **PPM software will drive change.**

What Are the Benefits of Project and Portfolio Management Software? What Are the Risks?

Gartner Research has found that the benefits of using a PPM system include, but are not limited to, the following (Stang 2006a, 16–17):

- "Significantly higher resource use rates.
- "Project sourcing based on access to a real-time resource pool. In this scenario, the project manager does not need to be familiar with the named resource but instead can find named resources based on skill sets and seek approval from the resource's manager to use the resource on a project.
- "Enhanced project actuals collection and comparisons to project estimates, both in terms of time and cost.
- "Real-time visibility into resource capacity versus inbound project demand.

- "Real-time, accurate scoping and assessment of the ability of an organization to handle and execute a project in terms of time, cost, and resources.
- "Identification of recurring skills shortages in the resource pool.
- "Communication of skills shortages to a human resources department for more effective and strategic recruiting.
- "Cost, time, and resource assessment of potential projects using outsourced labor, in-house labor, or a mix of both.
- "More accurate billing and invoicing of service projects to an external client or internal department (chargeback).
- "Enhanced project life cycle management, supporting all communication; work flow; and approval processes for scoping, sourcing, executing, and billing for a project.
- "Replacement of a series of manually intensive stand-alone tools, such as Microsoft Excel and other project-related point tools, with an integrated PPM suite.
- "Role-based support, allowing team contributors to work and add input into PM practices without requiring 'power user PM' skills.
- "Role-based support allowing project managers to more accurately see and report on project status.
- "Role-based support, allowing business development managers to view key project investments in high-level views and analyze these portfolios of projects in terms of earned value and ROI. It also allows these users to see the 'health' of projects at high levels.
- "'Operations' cost and resource tracking, as opposed to 'project' cost and resource tracking. Traditional PM tools could only track costs, resources, and work if a formal project plan was created. The latest PPM tools support all operations tracking in terms of time, cost, and resource use.
- "More efficient project delivery, including improved project execution based on on-time and on-budget success

factors, as well as proactive project rejection, postponement or cancellation based on real-world rationale."

But there are also risks. Some of those identified by Gartner
Research are (Stang 2006a, 17–18):

- "Project contributors and managers experiencing ongoing deadline and project work pressures can resist the
  adoption of newly introduced tools to their desktops out
  of fear that the learning curve of such tools could hinder
  their day-to-day productivity. Left to their own devices,
  these users sometimes have no choice but to rely on their
  own knowledge and management practices to get project
  work done. Resistance to newly added PPM tools could
  occur, so potential PPM tool customers should educate
  their project managers and contributors on how to use
  the tool to their benefit.
- "Best-of-breed (BOB) portfolio management tools—when
  used in stand-alone fashion—may require daily care on
  the administrator side to push data from key data sources
  to the analytical tools for effective analysis. When investing in a BOB portfolio management tool, the customer
  must understand that internal resources and data management are required to meet to get the stand-alone itera-
  tions of these tools to work effectively.
- "The PPM market is under intense consolidation. Potential PPM customers should consider vendor viability to
  ensure that their investment in a tool is secured with the
  vendor for at least five years. Hasty investments in PPM
  tools could lead to lack of support or product innovations
  if a vendor is selected and then acquired or goes out of
  business due to market conditions, a difficult economic
  period, or other financial and economic factors."

Stand-Alone Desktop versus Enterprise Software

Many of the advantages of enterprise products are the result
of using a single, central database. Because enterprise products

use a single server to store data, they eliminate the problem of having outdated data on multiple stand-alone computers. All users have access to and update the same databases, so everyone has access to the same information, facilitating communication and avoiding errors and wasted time involved when people are looking at different versions of the same data. Access to all available information also allows the user to determine, for example, whether staff are available to work on a project and what their skills and location are. Conversely, staff who are not fully utilized can be identified.

> Many of the advantages of enterprise products are the result of using a single, central database. Because enterprise products use a single server to store data, they eliminate the problem of having outdated data on multiple stand-alone computers.

Gartner Research refers to enterprise products as project and portfolio management because they aggregate information to create a view of the portfolio of projects in the organization (Stang 2006a).

"Portfolio management," according to Daniel Stang, author of *Project and Portfolio Management Applications,* "refers to the ongoing management of projects in a pipeline and projects in the midst of execution. Whereas traditional project management refers to single-project planning, project portfolio management adds the real-world pipeline and resource views based on utilization (booked), availability (capacity, not booked), inbound demand (project requests), and existing inventory (committed projects and projects in execution mode). Users can staff projects in the pipeline as resources become available, enabling planning above the single-project view" (Stang 2006a, 10).

Gartner Research further distinguishes between portfolio management and *portfolio analysis.* "Portfolio analysis focuses on the process of prioritizing high-level initiatives and their respective programs and projects, using algorithms and measurements to predict value, such as time-phased ROI. It is possible to perform ongoing portfolio analysis (and many different types of organizations do this) without investing in a full-blown PPM system" (Stang 2006a, 10).

The views offered by products that support portfolio management can also be used to prioritize projects. "Project portfolio management functions can roll up information about groups of projects to views that roles other than 'project manager' can understand. The views provide a form of communication between business management of an enterprise and the underlying IT department supporting the business-enabling technologies and systems for operations" (Stang 2006a, 11).

Portfolio management and project management tools may be sold as separate modules. The interest of an organization in either may depend on the current status of project management. Organizations with multiple projects that are not interested in enforcing a standard project management methodology may purchase a portfolio management module first. Organizations concerned about uniformity in project management could purchase the project management module first and then implement portfolio management when the data on all projects become available. Current project size, risk, and resistance to central control could be the determining factors.

What Are the Major Differences between Enterprise Products?

Advanced features include "ERP (Enterprise Resource Planning) integration, 3rd party project import from a variety of PPM vendors, advanced portfolio management features such as 'What If' modeling, and support for customization using third generation language tools such as Microsoft-Visual Studio and Java integrated development environments" (Quinn 2005).

Phased Implementation

Using PPM software requires the automation of processes, placing demands on staff. New data will have to be collected and used, and new skills must be learned. To help in the transition, PPM software can be acquired in phases.

"One type would include deploying time reporting and building out a resource skills database first and perhaps selecting a set number of key projects to track, adding them to the system. Another type of approach would include starting at the portfolio level, inputting an inventory of a set number of projects into the portfolio system, and adding some high-level resource information to the portfolio for identifying constraints, bottlenecks and hidden capacity vs. demand issues that potentially could put projects in the mix at risk if new projects are added" (Stang 2006b, 3). Organizations that adopt a phased approach can buy software in modules or use a vendor that is a software as a service (SAAS) or on-demand provider.

What an Organization Can Expect to Pay

Single-desktop software ranges in price from free (e.g., Computer Associates' Open Workbench; www.openworkbench. org) to hundreds of dollars per user license. Microsoft Project Standard is the market leader for desktop applications, but it is being challenged by other products (Essex 2006).

Enterprise software is more expensive. Licenses have to be purchased for more users. Fees can vary according to role, with the most expensive licenses for project managers and the least expensive for viewing reports. SAAS or on-demand products can be less expensive.

> There is a considerable difference in cost for a PPM system when comparing the SAAS option to a full PPM implementation. License-based PPM deals charge per module (between $25,000 and $50,000 per module), a server fee (varies based on whether or not the server fee includes all modules or if modules are listed separately "a la carte"), and role-based user fees for executive or portfolio manager ($2,400), project/ resource manager ($800 to $1,800) and team member ($150 to $300). Maintenance fees also apply. For a SAAS option, the cost could be as low as $20 per user per month. Using a SAAS PPM vendor can allow a smaller organization to spend less money on automation of process and more on creating and adopting better ones. (Stang 2006b, 5)

eProject's PPM6 is priced at $45 per user per month as a SAAS. Installed server licenses are also available for an additional one-time server fee of $15,000 (eProject 2006).

It is important to remember that implementation of PPM software will rarely involve just automating an existing project management process. It is likely to be part of the implementation of significant changes in project management, both because of a need for improving performance and to leverage the new capabilities offered by the software. The true costs are likely to be incurred over a period of time. "Potential customers of PPM applications need to visualize PPM as an investment in process and tools. The investment should include a budget for both sides, so that project organizations evaluate, change and adopt new and existing PPM processes and then automate these processes as they become stable and used widely in the organization" (Stang 2006a, 19–20).

User Acceptance

Some of the biggest failures in PPM software implementation are "a result of little end-user acceptance because of insufficient training, the perception that the application is being forced on end users and the absence of champions among peers" (Mohrmann and Kropf 2007, 36). Implementation should be managed like any significant change in how work is done. It would be a mistake to view PPM software as only requiring the training and involvement of IT staff. Leadership is required by senior management, and users need to be adequately trained and involved in planning the implementation.

An implementation team should be formed that includes the CIO, the PPM system project manager, the vendor project manager, and the person who will support the application when it is implemented. A project manager user group should be formed as well as an executive steering committee that includes key business unit leaders and the CIO (Mohrmann and Kropf 2007, 35).

Resources

The Project Management Institute (www.pmi.org) offers training, publications, and certification in project management. Members can join a health care project management special interest group.

Gartner Research (www.gartner.com) offers publications and other services on IT topics.

The Project Management Center (www.infogoal.com/pmc/pmchome.htm) aggregates information on project management, including training and software. It includes the Project Management Software Library (www.infogoal.com/pmc/pmcswr.htm).

Gantthead.com (www.gantthead.com) calls itself the "online community for IT project managers" and offers articles, news, and discussions.

Project Reference (www.projectreference.com) is a site maintained by John Musser at Columbia University. It includes course syllabi and class notes as well as suggested books and readings.

The International Institute for Learning (www.iil.com/pm) offers training and publications on project management. It maintains allPM.com (www.allpm.com), "the project manager's homepage."

Project Perfect offers a series of white papers on topics concerning project management (www.projectperfect.com.au/wp_index.php).

References
for Chapters 4–6

Berkun, Scott. 2005. *The art of project management.* Sebastopol, CA: O'Reilly Media.

eProject. 2006. EProject OnDemand PPM takes hold in healthcare industry. June 5. http://www.eproject.com/document_library/PR_Healthcare. pdf?doc=DL&ind=Healthcare (accessed May 8, 2007).

Essex, David E. 2006. Open-Workbench: Microsoft Project killer? *PM Network,* June. http://www.openworkbench.org/images/stories/Articles/ pmi-open-workbench.pdf (accessed May 8, 2007).

Garton, Colleen. 2004. *Fundamentals of technology project management.* Lewisville, TX: MC Press Online.

Isola, Miriam, Audrius Polikaitis, and Rose Ann Laureto. 2006. Implementation of a project management office (PMO)—Experiences from year 1. *Journal of Healthcare Information Management* 20 (1): 79–87.

Light, Matt, Matthew Hotle, Daniel B. Stang, and Jack Heine. 2005. *Project management office: The IT control tower.* Gartner Research No. G00132836. Stamford, CT: Gartner Research.

Meyer, N. Dean. 2005. Understanding the project management office. *CIO Magazine,* September 26. http://www.cio.com/article/12263/ understanding_the_project_management_office (accessed May 8, 2007).

Mohrmann, Gregg, and Roger Kropf. 2007. IT management and governance systems and their emergence in healthcare. *Journal of Healthcare Information Management* 21 (1): 33–39. http://www.himss.org/content. files/08_focus_ITMgmt.pdf (accessed May 8, 2007).

Pickens, Scott, and Jamie Solak. 2005. Successful healthcare programs and projects: Organization portfolio management essentials. *Journal of Healthcare Information Management* 19 (1): 19–27.

Project Management Institute. 2004. *Guide to the project management body of knowledge.* 3rd ed. Newtown Square, PA: Project Management Institute.

Quinn, Evan. 2005. A case for on-demand project and portfolio management. IDC. http://www.eproject.com/document_library/IDC_ wp.pdf?doc=DL&ind=IT (accessed May 8, 2007).

Richardson, Gary L., and Charles W. Butler. 2006. *Readings in information technology project management.* Boston: Thomson Course Technology.

Santosus, Megan. 2003. Office discipline: Why you need a project management office. *CIO Magazine,* July 1. http://www.cio.com/article/29887/ Why_You_Need_a_Project_Management_Office_PMO_ (accessed May 8, 2007).

Schwalbe, Kathy. 2006. *Information technology project management.* 4th ed. Boston: Thomson Course Technology.

Standish Group International, Inc. 2001. *Extreme CHAOS.* http://www. smallfootprint.com/Portals/0/Standish%20Group%20-%20Extreme%20 Chaos%202001.pdf (accessed May 7, 2007).

Stang, Daniel B. 2006a. *Project and portfolio management applications: Perspective.* Gartner Research No. G00138176. Stamford, CT: Gartner Research.

———. 2006b. *When evaluating PPM vendors, include SAAS and on-demand options.* Gartner Research No. G00137467. Stamford, CT: Gartner Research.

Ware, Lorraine Cosgrove. 2003. Best practices for project management offices. *CIO Research Reports,* July 2. http://www2.cio.com/research/ surveyreport.cfm?id=58 (accessed July 17, 2006).

Weill, Peter, and Jeanne Ross. 2004. *IT governance: How top performers manage IT decision rights for superior results.* Boston: Harvard Business School Press.

Yourdon, Edward. 2004. *Death march.* 2nd ed. Upper Saddle River, NJ: Pearson Education.

Appendix

Summary of Other Project Management Knowledge Areas

OTHER PROJECT management knowledge areas include project quality management, project human resource management, project risk management, and project procurement management.

Project Quality Management

Project Quality Management includes the processes and activities of the performing organization that determine quality policies, objectives, and responsibilities so that the project will satisfy the needs for which it was undertaken. It implements the quality management system through policy and procedures, with continuous process improvement activities conducted throughout, as appropriate. The Project Quality Management processes include:

- Quality Planning—identifying which quality standards are relevant to the project and determining how to satisfy them
- Perform Quality Assurance—applying the planned, systematic quality activities to ensure that the project employs all processes needed to meet requirements
- Perform Quality Control—monitoring specific project results to determine whether they comply with relevant quality standards, and identifying ways to eliminate causes of unsatisfactory performance

Source: Project Management Institute. 2004. *A Guide to the Project Management Body of Knowledge (PMBOK® Guide)*, 3rd ed., appendix F. Copyright and all rights reserved. Material from this publication has been reproduced with permission of the Project Management Institute.

Project Human Resource Management

Project Human Resource Management includes the processes that organize and manage the project team. The project team is comprised of the people who have assigned roles and responsibilities for completing the project. While it is common to speak of roles and responsibilities being assigned, team members should be involved in much of the project's planning and decision making. Early involvement of team members adds expertise during the planning process and strengthens commitment to the project. The type and number of project team members can often change as the project progresses. Project team members can be referred to as the project's staff. Project Human Resource Management processes include:

- Human Resource Planning—Identifying and documenting project roles, responsibilities, and reporting relationships, as well as creating the staffing management plan
- Acquire Project Team—Obtaining the human resources needed to complete the project
- Develop Project Team—Improving the competencies and interaction of team members to enhance project performance
- Manage Project Team—Tracking team member performance, providing feedback, resolving issues, and coordinating changes to enhance project performance

Project Risk Management

Project Risk Management includes the processes concerned with conducting risk management planning, identification, analysis, responses, and monitoring and control on a project. The objectives of Project Risk Management are to increase the probability and impact of positive events and decrease the probability and impact of events adverse to project objectives. Project Risk Management processes include:

- Risk Management Planning—deciding how to approach, plan, and execute the risk management activities for a project
- Risk Identification—determining which risks might affect the project, and documenting their characteristics
- Qualitative Risk Analysis—prioritizing risks for subsequent further analysis or action by assessing and combining their probability of occurrence and impact
- Quantitative Risk Analysis—numerically analyzing the effect on overall project objectives of identified risks
- Risk Response Planning—developing options and actions to enhance opportunities and to reduce threats to project objectives
- Risk Monitoring and Control—tracking identified risks, monitoring residual risks, identifying new risks, executing risk response plans, and evaluating their effectiveness throughout the project life cycle

Project Procurement Management

Project Procurement Management includes the processes to purchase or acquire the products, services, or results needed from outside the project team to perform the work. This chapter presents two perspectives of procurement. The organization can be either the buyer or seller of the product, service, or results under a contract.

Project Procurement Management includes the contract management and change control processes required to administer contracts or purchase orders issued by authorized project team members. Project Procurement Management also includes administering any contract issued by an outside organization (the buyer) that is acquiring the project from the performing organization (the seller) and administering contractual obligations placed on the project team by the contract. Project Procurement Management processes include:

- Plan Purchases and Acquisitions—determining what to purchase or acquire, and determining when and how
- Plan Contracting—documenting products, services, and results requirements, and identifying potential sellers
- Request Seller Responses—obtaining information, quotations, bids, offers, or proposals, as appropriate
- Select Sellers—reviewing offers, choosing from among potential sellers, and negotiating a written contract with a seller
- Contract Administration—managing the contract and the relationship between the buyer and the seller, reviewing and documenting how a seller is performing or has performed to establish required corrective actions and provide a basis for future relationships with the seller, managing contract-related changes and, when appropriate, managing the contractual relationship with the outside buyer of the project
- Contract Closure—completing and settling each contract, including the resolution of any open items, and closing each contract

PART III

Performance Management after Implementation

Introduction

Part III explores what should happen after an information technology (IT) implementation. How can an organization find out if it got the benefits that were expected—and increase the chances of success the next time? We describe how a post-implementation audit can be carried out by comparing pre- and post-implementation performance, conducting time and motion studies, and studying pilot installations.

What can organizations do to get the benefits that were expected? Value is not automatically received because the project is completed and works as planned. Information technology that produces labor savings does not necessarily result in fewer staff and lower labor costs or in current staff redirecting their time to another valuable activity. Having defined benefits at the beginning, managers need to ensure that benefits are received at the end. This requires the identification of the expected benefits, a plan for achieving them, and an analysis of what was actually obtained.

Formal benefits realization processes that seek to define and manage the attainment of benefits are described. This often involves the creation of special teams and the definition of who is accountable for achieving each benefit. Some organizations have developed a written contract called a service level agreement (SLA) with an external vendor or an internal IT department. We define SLAs and how they can be negotiated and used internally. We consider the possible positive and negative effects of SLAs, how they can be measured, and what costs are involved.

What All Hospitals Should Be Doing

Post-Implementation Audits

Do a post-implementation audit to determine if the expected benefits are received.

Benefits Realization

Aggressively go after the benefits.

1. Assign someone the responsibility to get them. Evaluate that person on whether the benefits are gained.

2. Support those being held accountable. Create teams with the knowledge and resources to define the benefits, measure their achievement, and help those accountable produce the changes in processes and staff behavior that will be needed.

Service Level Agreements

1. Use SLAs regardless of whether the hospital outsources IT or uses internal staff.

2. Meet with managers and users to define and agree on the SLAs. Continue to change SLAs, raising the target or eliminating them if they are regularly achieved or adding new ones.

3. Develop a contract that includes SLAs.

4. Performance evaluation of the IT department and the chief information officer should be based at least in part on the achievement of SLAs.

Customer Satisfaction Surveys

Customer satisfaction surveys should be conducted regularly for all the components of IT.

Decisions

Health care managers need to make a number of decisions, which can be facilitated by answering the following questions.

Post-Implementation Audits

Do we need to do an audit? Without an audit, you will not know if you got the benefits that were cited to justify the expense. Even more important is the information that will be gained on what elements of the project produced benefits. Information technology investments are made year after year, so the benefits from next year's projects may be lost by not understanding what did not work.

Without data from before the implementation, what do we do? While a pre-implementation study would be ideal, many organizations do not do one. You then need to decide how much time and money to spend. The choices are:

- Use existing records, both manual and computerized. Some of these data will have to be labor intensive to recover. The data needed to document all of the important benefits may not be available.
- Compare facilities with and without the IT. The facilities to be compared need to be selected carefully to help ensure that those differences do not explain the changes observed. Some adjustments in the data can be made when the calculations are done (e.g., case-mix adjustment).

Focus on the benefits that are most critical for future investments because they save money or increase revenue, improve quality, or increase executive or staff acceptance.

Benefits Realization

Can we get benefits without a formal "realization" process? Many benefits are not achieved automatically, especially where people are affected. A reduction in manual paper completion does not automatically result in the departure of the people who handled the paper. Nor do those people, by themselves, redirect their efforts to activities that provide the most value to the organization. Benefits need to be managed, and the basic elements of management need to be applied—including making someone accountable, developing a plan of action, setting a timeline, measuring achievement, and providing incentives.

How can we make staff accountable for getting benefits? People cannot be held accountable unless they are formally assigned responsibility, are given the resources they need, and know they will be asked to report back. This can be done as part of the budgeting process, during which an "owner" or "sponsor" of the project can be defined. It can be part of an annual personnel review process in which staff define goals and report on performance. An important consideration is defining ownership. If all projects involving IT are considered to belong to the IT department, then other managers, staff, and clinicians cannot be held accountable for success or failure. Joint or sole accountability of the owner or sponsor has to be defined. Senior management needs to assign accountability and take the time to determine what benefits were received.

Service Level Agreements

Should we be using SLAs? With just external vendors or internally? Service level agreements are important for setting expectations and replacing attitudes and anecdotes with empirical data. Saying "IT never delivers" or "I don't have what I need to get my work done" is not acceptable. Service level agreements quantify what the users can expect and allow the IT provider to be held accountable. Accountability and performance are as important for an internal IT department as they are for an outsourced provider. Service level agreements are helpful because they compel their customers to define their expectations.

Can managers and users really define SLAs? Aren't they technical—about the performance of the hardware and software? Who should write them? Service level agreements that are important to the user should be included, such as the availability of applications vital to their work. Users should be involved in writing SLAs so that their expectations are met and they begin to understand the cost of providing the level of service they want. Service level agreements about the performance of hardware and software should be included when they are directly related to getting users the services they want.

Are there other reasons to write SLAs besides saving money? Other compelling reasons to write SLAs include regulatory compliance, patient safety, quality, and the need to meet or exceed the performance of competitors.

What level of management needs to be involved? The manager who is one level up from the unit whose performance is affected needs to be involved. An SLA concerning the delivery of lab results will be monitored by the director of the lab, but the manager in charge of ancillary services also needs to be involved. Managers need to know what the SLAs are, monitor them, and be involved in decisions about performance improvement. This level of participation helps ensure that the process is taken seriously.

7

Post-Implementation Audits

A POST-IMPLEMENTATION audit (PIA) is a study of what benefits were received from a project, as well as the actual costs. Organizations do have reasons not to do such an audit. It takes time just when work may be returning to normal after implementation, and it may reveal that the benefits that justified the investment were not achieved. But PIAs are important. "PIAs provide a thorough approach for proving the value of high-cost, mission-critical IT investments and for gleaning project management best practices, which [chief information officers (CIOs)] can then apply to keep subsequent projects on track" (Levinson 2003).

Post-implementation audits can also reveal patterns, such as problems arising whenever a particular type of application is installed or when the installation involves a particular unit of the organization.

To overcome the reluctance to do an audit, organizations can make it the last step in the project plan and part of the project management and governance process. University Hospitals in Cleveland (see the case study following the introduction to this book) requires project sponsors to return after implementation and set side by side the benefits that were predicted and what actually occurred.

> To overcome the reluctance to do an audit, organizations can make it the last step in the project plan and part of the project management and governance process.

Audits should be carried out by a team that consists of a manager or clinician from the unit that sponsored the project and the IT person involved in the implementation. The sponsor can "more easily determine if an external factor rather than a systems failure is causing a system to not generate expected value" (Levinson 2003), while someone from IT will understand the technology. The team should also include staff members not involved in the implementation, including someone from the finance department.

A number of different methodologies are available for carrying out an audit. Table 7-1 summarizes the strengths of the three methods described below. Considerations in selecting a method are discussed at the end of this chapter.

Comparing Pre- and Post-Implementation Performance

Badger, Bosch, and Toteja (2005) carried out a post-implementation return on investment (ROI) analysis of the implementation of an electronic health record (EHR) at the George Washington University Medical Faculty Associates (MFA), a multispecialty physician practice in Washington, DC.

"A high-level, very conservative return-on-investment analysis" conducted by MFA four months after rollout revealed a 35 percent reduction in daily paper chart pulls following the EHR implementation for an estimated annual reduction of 144,083 pulls. Based on an average cost of $5.66 in chart-room staff time for each chart pull, MFA estimated a first-year savings of $81,551. When RN time devoted to chart responsibilities was factored in, the first-year savings on decreased chart pulls were estimated to be $335,900 (Badger, Bosch, and Toteja 2005).

Table 7-1. Strengths of Three Post-Implementation Audit Methods

Pre-/Post-Implementation	Demonstrates actual changes in a specific facility
Time/Motion	Accurate data on the time required to complete a task to address staff and clinician concerns
Study Pilots	Does not require pre-implementation data

Revenues were also affected by the new system, "thanks largely to more accurate reimbursement coding generated by the EHR's built-in documentation templates." Medical Faculty Associates estimated that its physicians were undercoding 9 percent of patient visits before using the EHR, resulting in a reimbursement loss of $695,877 per year. Based on a 30 percent first-year reduction in "downcoding," MFA estimates that the EHR would eliminate improper coding by the end of the third year of the implementation. Further reductions in transcription expenses ($1.3 million over five years) and the costs of developing new patient charts ($1.23 million) bring the total estimated positive financial impact of the EHR to more than $11.7 million over five years (Badger, Bosch, and Toteja 2005, 39–40).

The Massachusetts Technology Collaborative and New England Healthcare Institute (2006) commissioned a study by First Consulting Group of hospitals that had implemented computerized physician order entry (CPOE). Five hospitals were selected using the following criteria:

- CPOE is used in more than 80 percent of the hospital units.
- At least 75 percent of orders are entered by physicians using CPOE.
- More than 50 percent of admissions are managed by independent community physicians.

The key points discovered by this research related to the assessment of benefits were (Massachusetts Technology Collaborative and New England Healthcare Institute 2006, 9):

- Study hospitals did not have the resources to do much pre-CPOE measurement requiring manual data collection, so they tended to rely on metrics already collected for other purposes.
- System reports concerning the incidence and responses to clinical decision support (e.g., drug, allergy checking) and the use of institutional order sets not only demonstrate

value but also aid in efforts to improve the effectiveness of clinical decision support.

• All hospitals were able to obtain system reports on physician use of CPOE and used these to target physicians for additional support or encouragement.

Table 7-2 shows the impact metrics used by these hospitals and in studies found in the literature and the sources of information. While many of the measures required the manual extraction of data, two hospitals were able to measure "physician response to CPOE order reminders/alerts" by examining system reports showing how often alerts, such as drug-drug interaction or lab test duplication, are fired (sent to the physician to appear on the screen) and how often physicians change or cancel an order in response. All hospitals took advantage of system reports that showed how often physicians used CPOE. These reports allowed the hospital to target physicians who used CPOE less frequently for follow-up training and/or counseling.

"Study hospitals that were able to obtain pre-post metrics demonstrated significant improvements in order management. For example, one hospital had radiology and laboratory turnaround time for orders collapse from 1 hour to 10–15 minutes. This hospital also experienced a 50 percent reduction in pharmacist calls to physicians for order clarification. In another hospital, calls to physicians from pharmacy dropped 77 percent and the turnaround time for radiology orders by 50 percent. Similarly, the average time lag from medication order to administration was reduced from 90 minutes to 11 minutes" (Massachusetts Technology Collaborative and New England Healthcare Institute 2006, 11).

Time and Motion Studies

Some pre- and post-implementation studies utilize information obtained from existing records or automated systems. Studies conducted this way may not provide information on the time spent carrying out tasks, however. Existing human resource systems may not require staff to enter detailed information on

Table 7-2. Computerized Physician Order Entry in Community Hospitals—Impact Metrics

Impact Metrics and Sources of Information	
Lag time from order to administration of STAT med	Manual study (order time available from CPOE for the "after study;" admin time from e-MAR—electronic Medication Administration Record—if in place before CPOE)
Lag time from order to administration of antibiotic	Manual study (order time available from CPOE for the "after study;" admin time from e-MAR if in place before CPOE)
Lag time from medication order to administration (overall)	Manual study (order time available from CPOE for the "after study;" admin time from e-MAR if in place before CPOE)
Laboratory test turnaround time	Manual study in pre; data extraction from system in post
Errors resulting from order transcription	Manual study
Length of stay	Analysis of Admission/Discharge/Transfer data
Medication-related errors and adverse drug events	Generally tracked based on incident reporting and surveillance
Pharmacist telephone calls to clarify medical orders	Manual logging
Order changes following pharmacist review/verification	Manual logging
Pharmacist time devoted to medication order verification	Manual study aided by extraction of some system data
Lag time for pharmacist verification of medication orders	Manual study aided by extraction of some system data
Verbal orders not signed within required time	Manual study; may be routinely tracked
Physician response to CPOE order reminders/alerts (order is changed) • Medication alerts • Medication substitution • Switch to oral from IV • Lab duplicate checking • Radiology duplicate checking	Post only; only if system can track and report on incidence of, and response to, alerts
Inappropriate medication or route	Manual study in pre; extraction of data from system in post study
Compliance with JCAHO standard for orders for restraints	Manual study in pre; extraction of data from system in post study
Compliance with care recommendations in Core Measures	Manual study in pre; extraction of data from system in post study (data typically already collected for reporting)

Source: Reprinted with permission from *Computerized Physician Order Entry: Lessons Learned from Community Hospitals,* published by the Massachusetts Technology Collaborative and the New England Healthcare Institute. Copyright © 2006.

the time spent on activities. Further, paper medical records may not provide detailed or reliable data. More accurate data on the time required to complete a task can be determined by a time and motion study. Observers follow clinicians and record how long specific tasks, such as entering an order or charting the administration of a drug, take to complete. These studies can be used to measure improvements in efficiency. The amount of time that is saved can then be used to calculate the financial impact of the application.

Researchers at Partners HealthCare in Boston (www.partners.org) have created a Microsoft Access database to help observers record time and motion data and store them for analysis. A user's guide is also available as well as a journal article that provides a case example of how the tool can be used (Pizziferri et al. 2005). The tool and supporting documents can be downloaded for free by going to http://healthit.ahrq.gov and entering "EHR Time & Motion Tool" in the Search box.

Pizziferri and colleagues (2005) conducted a time-motion study in primary care clinics of Partners HealthCare System. They wanted to know if implementation of an EHR increased the time required for physicians to do their work and whether it affected the time physicians spend in direct patient care. Post-implementation, the adjusted mean overall time spent per patient during clinic sessions decreased by 0.5 minutes, from a pre-intervention adjusted average of 27.55 minutes to a post-intervention adjusted average of 27.05 minutes. No significant change (13.3 minutes versus 13.6 minutes) was seen in the time spent in direct patient care after EHR implementation. While a majority of physicians responding to the survey believed EHR use results in quality improvement, only 29 percent reported that EHR documentation takes the same amount of time or less compared to the paper-based system (Pizziferri et al. 2005, 176).

Mekhjian et al. (2002) conducted a time-motion study in a dedicated surgical organ transplant unit at the Ohio State University Medical Center following implementation of CPOE.

They found a 64 percent reduction in medication turnaround time from 5 hours, 28 minutes (before CPOE) to 1 hour, 51 minutes (after CPOE). "The two key phases that saw improvement were communication of the order to pharmacy (which includes the steps between physician ordering and dispensing by pharmacy) and administration of the dispensed medication to the patient (which includes the steps between dispensing by pharmacy and administration of the medication to the patient). The first phase decreased from 3 hours, 57 minutes to 33 minutes, and the second phase decreased from 3 hours, 16 minutes to 1 hour, 22 minutes" (Mekhjian et al. 2002, 534).

Taylor, Manzo, and Sinnett (2002) at Montefiore Medical Center (www.montefiore.org) conducted a time-motion study before and after CPOE implementation and used the results to determine cost savings. They found that ward clerks each saved 120 minutes per day after CPOE replaced the paper medication ordering process. Nurses each saved about 20 minutes per day (Taylor, Manzo, and Sinnett 2002, 45).

The value of time-motion studies is that they provide evidence of actual changes in behavior, which supplements the perceptions of users about what has occurred. This does not mean that perceptions are not important. Time-motion studies can help managers and users understand whether changes are needed in applications or how they are being implemented, for example, the need for increased user support or training. Such studies can also isolate the steps in a complex process that are most responsible for overall changes and that highlight the remaining bottlenecks. They can also provide the basis for estimating reductions in operating expenses.

Using Studies of Pilot Installations

While many studies compare data from pre- to post-implementation, other methods are available. An area undergoing a pilot implementation can be compared to areas still using existing technology or paper records.

Ohio State University Medical Center

Mekhjian et al. (2002, 535), studying CPOE implementation at the Ohio State University Medical Center, compared two surgical and medical intensive care units with and without CPOE that were comparable in terms of patient population and acuity. Comparison of laboratory turnaround times for the two units revealed a 25 percent reduction in result reporting time. The average result reporting time in the surgical intensive care unit (ICU) using CPOE was 23 minutes, 4 seconds. In the medical ICU, where manual order entry was used, the result reporting time was 31 minutes, 3 seconds.

Banner Estrella Medical Center

Banner Estrella Medical Center (BEMC) is a 172-bed hospital that opened in Phoenix, Arizona, in February 2005 (see the case study at the end of part III). It is a new hospital in a new location, not a replacement facility. Banner Estrella Medical Center is a pilot site for what Banner Health calls *care transformation*—the combination of technology, process redesign, evidence-based best practices and the cultural transformation necessary to make the adoption successful. It utilizes enabling technology, such as electronic medical records (EMRs), automated alerts, and CPOE.

Together, staff from Banner Health, Cerner, and Intel examined data relating to key performance indicators from January to June 2006, the most recent period for which data was available. They used the Intel Healthcare IT Economic Model (www.intel.com/healthcare/healthit). The benefits study was done to sustain the momentum as care transformation is rolled out across the other facilities. Banner Health also needed to know if care transformation is working before it is replicated for all hospitals. Improvements can also be made in the systems operating at BEMC, and new features are piloted there before they are rolled out to other facilities.

Because they could not conduct a pre- and post-implementation analysis of a new hospital, the team compared BEMC to a "virtual hospital" based on the weighted average of eight Banner Health hospitals that had not implemented care transformation. The team looked at ten key indicators and identified up to $2.8 million in financial benefits for the six-month period by calculating the difference between BEMC and the virtual hospital. The analysis showed:

- Lower average length of stay
- Lower overtime expenditure per 1,000 admissions
- Lower drug expenditure per 1,000 adjusted admissions (adjusted for case mix)
- Lower form expenditure per 1,000 admissions
- Lower document storage costs per 1,000 admissions
- Greater avoidance of costs for treating adverse drug events (ADEs) per 1,000 acute admissions
- Fewer medical insurance claims per 1,000 acute admissions
- Fewer days in the accounts receivable department
- Fewer nurses leaving voluntarily within the first year of employment
- More emergency department visitors treated (because fewer patients left without treatment)

Case-mix adjustment was used to attempt to compensate for differences in the types of patients seen. Adjusting for case mix and considering only bottom-line impact, the benefits were estimated to be $1.3 million for the six-month period or $2.7 million annually.

The benefits study was undertaken to estimate the benefits from care transformation at BEMC. Other Banner facilities may see higher or lower benefits. A major risk in extrapolating the results at BEMC to other Banner hospitals is whether physicians will utilize CPOE, a requirement for obtaining medical staff membership at BEMC. Transitioning away from the paper chart may also have to happen incrementally because of the comfort level of staff with using paper; thus, the benefits may be achieved more slowly.

Selecting a Method

A pre- and post-implementation audit provides information on the benefits received at a specific facility. The most common problem in using this method is that data are not collected before implementation, making comparison impossible. This problem can be partially solved by searching for data that were routinely collected for other purposes before implementation. For example, the number of charts pulled may be collected routinely for the purpose of determining the efficiency of workers or to justify budget submissions. Computers also routinely collect information, some of which may be stored but never looked at. This could include the number of medications ordered by physicians before the implementation of CPOE.

Organizations may also want to collect data before implementation but do not have the money to invest in data collection, especially when very few processes are computerized. Data collection may require costly chart reviews or tabulations of data from paper records.

Organizations that want proof that specific changes occurred at facilities and are willing to bear the cost (or have existing systems in place that routinely collect data) should undertake a pre- and post-implementation audit.

Time and motion studies should be selected when organizations are particularly concerned about the effect of IT on the level of staff effort, especially when physicians and nurses are involved. Clinicians will be very concerned that new systems add to the work they have to do or do not reduce their work enough to justify the cost. For example, does a CPOE system increase the time required for ordering, and does that decrease over time? Does a medication system that utilizes a computer and bar-code scanner increase the time required by nurses? As noted earlier, an existing human resource or medical record system may not provide such detailed data on the time required for specific tasks. Time and motion studies can yield accurate data. The cost will be justified when clinician acceptance is a significant issue.

Comparing a pilot to an existing organization can provide information when pre-implementation data are unavailable. Rather than using published data from unfamiliar organizations to determine benefits, the pilot organization can be compared to known facilities in the same system or community. This method can benefit both the pilot and the organization to which it is being compared. The pilot can gain a greater understanding of what changes have occurred, while the other organization can gain some understanding of what benefits it might achieve. The objection to this method will be that the two facilities are different and the comparison is invalid. This concern might be reduced by selecting comparable facilities and by adjusting the data for known differences, such as case mix. One methodology is described in the BEMC case study at the end of part III.

8

Benefits Realization

VALUE IS NOT automatically received because the project is completed and works as planned. Information technology that produces labor savings does not necessarily result in fewer staff and lower labor costs, or current staff redirecting their time to another valuable activity. Formal benefits realization processes seek to define and manage the attainment of benefits. This often involves the creation of special teams and the definition of who is accountable for achieving each benefit.

Accountability and Ownership

Assigning accountability for achieving the benefits of a project is essential. This brings us back to the question of what an "IT project" is and who owns it. University Hospitals (UH) in Cleveland (see the case study following the introduction to this book) believes the IT department is the enabler but not the owner of projects, with the exception of IT infrastructure projects such as expansion or upgrade of computer storage. Even after becoming operational, the systems belong to the operating units. The IT department provides technical support such as hardware and network maintenance.

The governance process at UH is used to create and reinforce accountability by the business units for projects. The business-unit project sponsor presents the project to the IT advisory committee and the IT steering committee. University Hospitals has a "closed loop" governance process, dictating that, if the project is approved, the same sponsor must return six months to a year after the project goes operational to a meeting of the steering committee and present a report on the completed project that parallels the initial proposal (which is presented on one slide). A side-by-side comparison is presented of the cost, objectives, and start/end dates.

Ed Marx, University Hopitals's CIO, says, "Who should be singularly accountable for an application to run the [operating room (OR)]? Can IT affect the processes within the OR? No. Can IT tell people in the OR how to use the application right? No. Who can? It is really the head nurse in the OR who is the project sponsor. She is singularly accountable. We can give them the hardware and software, but at the end of the day we can't tell them how to operate their business."

Murphy (2002, 124–26) contends that organizations must view each project as a business change project with IT components. He emphasizes that "without clear accountability, the business value of IT investments cannot be fully realized," and he presents these recommendations for achieving the benefits from a project:

- The benefits for which the individual is accountable must be clearly defined, avoiding vague aspirations such as "successfully deliver."
- Accountabilities should be decided and agreed on at the investment appraisal stage, not during the implementation stage.
- A clear distinction must be made between IT and business accountabilities. Information technology must be accountable for successfully delivering the appropriate technologies, infrastructure, and technical support, but IT is not accountable for delivering business benefits. This is the responsibility of the relevant business managers.
- A change management procedure should be put in place. The project will change as time progresses, and staff will leave or be reassigned to the project.
- The management mind-set must be changed. The concept of thinking through the full realization process will not come easily to most senior managers.
- The accountable manager must be provided with adequate resources and authority to deliver the benefits.

- Accountability for the eventual results must be reinforced periodically, especially through informal contacts.

The governance process in place at UH explicitly follows the first four of these recommendations.

Benefits Realization for Enterprisewide Projects

Major projects like the implementation of an electronic medical record (EMR) involve many units of an organization. There is no one owner. Allina Hospitals and Clinics in Minneapolis dealt with this issue by establishing a benefits realization team when it began implementation in 2003 of an enterprisewide integrated information system with inpatient clinical documentation and orders, clinical decision support, and revenue cycle applications. Allina also faced the need to achieve benefits across the four larger hospitals and seven small regional hospitals in its system. "The benefits team is responsible for the development and timely reporting of implementation, process, and outcome metrics for the department directors and other local leaders to use to evaluate their performance in realizing expected system benefits. However, the leadership at the local hospitals and clinics are fully accountable for the benefits expected from the system" (Thompson et al. 2005, 60).

Individuals and operating groups with direct responsibility for benefits were identified and held accountable by inclusion of the achievement of benefits in their job success criteria and departmental and organizational budgets. Expected benefits were loaded into Allina's budgets through 2008.

The systemwide benefits team is charged with defining, designing, and facilitating the achievement of expected benefits. For example, "The medical records team members primarily are nurses who are assigned specific high-volume DRGs. They research and summarize practice for each DRG, develop a cross-walk of all current Allina order sets and develop potential order set models for a team of physicians, pharmacists, and other clinicians to review and modify" (Thompson et al. 2005, 57).

The team maintains an updated catalogue of anticipated benefits, including updated estimates of each benefit, descriptions of the system functionality, and changes that must occur to realize each benefit. The team works with system designers and builders to ensure the system incorporates all aspects needed to achieve expected benefits. Integrated benefits plans are developed for each major benefit area, including detailed tasks, time frames, responsible parties, approach to and organization of work, organizational structures, project charters, metrics, and calculation methods.

Allina has recognized that making managers and clinicians accountable for achieving benefits is not enough. They must be supported, just as project managers and a project management office (PMO) can support them during project implementation. But realizing benefits from clinical or financial management systems requires detailed knowledge, analysis, and planning that is different from the *Guide to the Project Management Body of Knowledge* described in part II. Specialists, including nurses and physicians, need to be involved more than in an advisory role.

Realizing Cost Savings

A number of specific challenges face organizations in realizing certain benefits. When harvesting salary expense, entire positions have to be eliminated to have true cost savings. Saving a little time over a number of positions never results in cost reduction. If entire positions cannot be eliminated, any savings can be counted as efficiency improvement (which could increase throughput and revenue) or quality-of-care improvement (because additional time to accomplish the remaining tasks results in fewer errors and improved job satisfaction).

Changing work flow and methodology is frequently the greatest impediment to benefits realization. People tend to work in the same way they have always worked and resist change. Installing a new computer application on top of an existing process will not in itself result in an ROI or care transformation. The process itself has to change as well as the behavior of people, who need to learn to work in a different way. This is often resisted by saying, "This is the way we've always done it." The inevitable learning curve must be climbed with any new system, requiring time and effort. This issue was largely avoided at BEMC (see the case study at the end of part III) because no existing methodologies were in place that had to be changed. It was a new facility, and the staff did not have to make significant changes while keeping the hospital running day to day.

No benefits will be accrued until the staff accept and use a new system and change the way they work. Benefits will also accrue slowly as the learning curve is climbed. Implementing CPOE, for example, necessitates data entry work by physicians. They have to develop keyboard skills or familiarity with the interface of a handheld device. It becomes necessary for physicians to know the specific name under which a drug is stored in the ordering database and to compute the proper dose. Their work flow is actually slowed down for a period of time until these skills are learned. When alerts are added to a CPOE system, such as those used at BEMC to avoid adverse drug events, it adds an extra step to read the alert and a mouse click to react to it. This also slows physicians down and has to be balanced against the positive effect of fewer ADEs.

Structured Reporting Tools: Scorecards and Dashboards

Implementation studies have a fixed beginning and end. An alternative to conducting studies is a scorecard or dashboard that is updated to provide information. Domalewski and Berger (2005) describe the picture archiving and communications system (PACS) dashboard—the Imaging Manager Desktop—that was created at Fairview Health Services in Minneapolis. The desktop is available to both local managers and corporate executives (Domalewski and Berger 2005). The key performance indicators that are tracked include:

- Emergency department (ED) turnaround time
- General turnaround time
- Film costs
- Imaging availability
- Operating margin
- Employee productivity
- Late charges

For example, employee productivity (as defined by exams per full-time equivalent [FTE]) is monitored on a monthly basis at the department level and at the level of each modality and is compared to a target.

Allina Hospitals and Clinics in Minneapolis has developed a benefits dashboard as part of the benefits realization process for its integrated information system. Detailed metrics have been developed for each of the major areas of potential benefit. Data collection for most of these metrics can be automated. For example, detailed benefits metrics for the emergency department include length of stay for ED admissions and outpatient visits, the percentage of patients who left without being seen, per-visit cost of magnetic resonance imaging and computed tomography head and abdomen scans, gross and net revenues per visit, transcription lines and costs per visit, ADE types and location by facility, unit secretary and billing specialist FTE, and time study of ED activities (Thompson et al. 2005, 60).

Figure 8-1 is from a dashboard project completed by Velōz Global Solutions for Maimonides Medical Center in Brooklyn, New York. It provides the leadership team with real-time access to information that allows the team to monitor trends among Maimonides's business lines.

Figure 8-1. Capacity Management Dashboard for Maimonides Medical Center

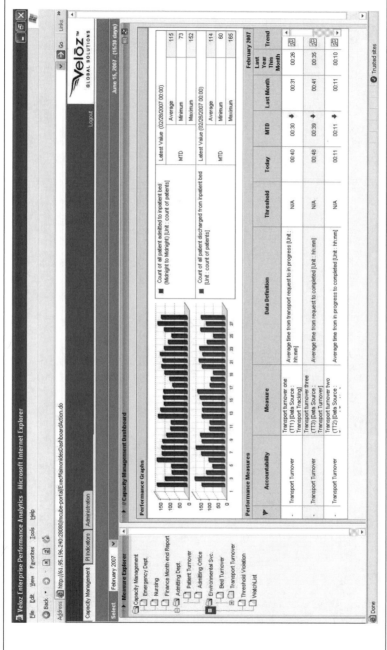

Source: Reprinted with permission from Maimonides Medical Center, Brooklyn, New York.

9

Service Level Agreements:
A Tool for Negotiating
and Sustaining Performance

Introduction

Service level agreements define standards of performance for essential IT services. Table 9-1 displays two SLAs in the contract between the University of Pennsylvania Health System (UPHS) and First Consulting Group (FCG). (See the University of Pennsylvania Health System case study at the end of part III.)

The SLA contract will stipulate a means to measure and report status and progress. Service level agreements often include a mechanism for addressing and improving poor performance, including financial penalties.

> Service level agreements can be used in situations when the IT department has entered into a contract with an external vendor, when IT has an agreement with an internal customer, and when an internal customer has chosen to sign an agreement with an external vendor directly.

To set expectations appropriately, it is important to make clear who are the customers and who are the providers. For example, the IT department may enter into an agreement with an internal unit, but delivery of the service actually depends on an external vendor. The internal unit should understand

---

Portions of this chapter were adapted from Session 5 at the Healthcare Information and Management Systems Society 2004 Annual Conference: Guy Scalzi and George Brenckle, "It's an IT Thing: The Importance of Measurement and SLAs."

Table 9-1. Sample Service Level Agreements

Service	Service Level	Service Metric	Metric Percentage
Support center/ Help desk	Help desk first call resolution	Resolution of calls at first contact that are within the scope of help desk staff resolution	65
	Answer time	Answered in less than thirty seconds	80

that and recognize that IT's role is to manage the vendor relationship. The IT department itself cannot guarantee delivery of the service. The ultimate provider may be an external vendor even when the agreement is between IT and the internal unit.

> **Service level agreements are the most important component in establishing performance expectations. They commit a service provider to a predetermined level of performance based on specific criteria.**

Service level agreements establish performance criteria on the front end of a relationship so that no surprises arise as the relationship progresses. Service level agreements can include penalties if performance criteria are not met. They are the mechanism or scorecard for monitoring ongoing performance and for driving a continuous improvement environment. They can vary on the basis of type of service and can drive pricing. Higher service levels command higher prices. Using objective measurement of IT services helps "substitute reality for subjective perception" (Garbani 2004, 9).

> **Service level agreements provide empirical data to replace stories—anecdotes about poor performance.**

Defining Service Level Agreements

Styles

Three different SLA styles are available for IT outsourcing:

1. Utility: Examples of IT business processes within the utility style include network, desktop, help desk, and data center. The basic measure is whether or not the service is acceptable or unacceptable. If the service is down, a credit is applied. An example would be 99.5 percent server availability.

2. Process improvement: This area measures the result of performance changes after the introduction of process refinements. It is used when the objective is process improvement following the service provider's assumption of responsibilities. An example would be that normal-priority dictionary[1] maintenance would be completed 99.5 percent of the time within 24 hours, with this metric met thirty days after the contract commencement date.

3. Value added: This type of SLA helps an organization describe the qualitative benefits they can reasonably expect to achieve in addition to quantifiable benefits. These SLAs measure the effectiveness in creating value for the organization. As an example, if the desired value is to attract and retain talent, the measured result would be the appropriate fit of the resources recruited and the duration of employment rather than how many people were recruited.

Categories

Service level agreements[2] can be divided into various categories, depending on the nature of the outsourcing relationship. For

---

[1]A data dictionary is a "database about data and databases. It holds the name, type, range of values, source, and authorization for access for each data element in the organization's files and databases. It also indicates which application programs use that data so that when a change in a data structure is contemplated, a list of affected programs can be generated" (TechWeb 2006).

[2]The term *service level agreement* is commonly used to describe the indicators, objectives, or targets that are included in the service level agreement itself.

IT outsourcing, the Application Service Provider (ASP) Industry Consortium divided key SLAs into four major categories, including:

1. Network: This covers the network connection between the customer and the ASP. The network service provider agrees on a suitable service level for delivery of Internet service provider (ISP) services. Possible metrics include availability, network latency (e.g., the time between initiating a request for data and the beginning of the actual data transfer), and low packet loss (i.e., the discarding of data packets—blocks of data—in a network when a device [switch, router, etc.] is overloaded and cannot accept any incoming data at a given moment) (TechWeb 2006).

2. Hosting: This covers the hosting services provided to the ASP. An ASP uses this type of agreement when hardware is hosted or co-located with a third party. Metrics vary, depending on the type of service, and could include service-order acknowledgment and mean time to respond.

3. Application: The ASP agrees to a certain level of responsibility, different class of service, performance parameters, and a manner of calculating both the demanded performance levels and penalties that result if the ASP does not perform as planned. "Application SLAs require the institution of application-specific metrics, that is, definitions of performance levels that relate to application utilization. For example, an application SLA should define the percent of user interactions, such as downloads or data requests, to be executed without failure. It should also define the acceptable time lapse between a user's request for data and the moment the updated data screen appears" (Carr 2001).

4. Customer care/help desk: These SLAs may specify how quickly a problem will be reported to customers after it has been identified and how quickly an identified problem will be resolved.

Major Elements

Service level agreements should include certain key elements:

- Purpose: what is the overall purpose of the measure (what is it trying to affect)?
- Description of service/duration: SLAs should articulate clearly what the service level is and how long it will be measured.
- Metrics: SLAs should include defined metrics (the exact goals or expectations).
- Payment and termination: SLAs should articulate payment terms and outline conditions for termination if performance measures are missed.

Characteristics

Service level agreements should also include certain key characteristics. They should be understandable by both parties, applicable, measurable, affordable, controllable, and agreeable. In essence, SLAs should not include any gray areas.

The client and supplier must understand the SLA. Simpler and more focused SLAs are desirable; vague or misleading SLAs serve no one, and clarity brings value to all parties. The measurement should be applicable. It should apply to what is being measured, correlate well with the customer's perception, and be something the service provider will change. Service level agreements only create value when they accurately represent service delivery in a given environment. This is not simple to accomplish. A measure like "low packet loss" is precise, but may not be understood by managers outside of IT. "Availability" and even "latency" are easier to understand, but neither measure reflects the same dimension of quality.

The service should be measured in a way that is consistent, and common measurement techniques should be used for all customers. The timeline for measurement should be coordinated with customer expectations. Performance should not be measured selectively, and measurement should be automated wherever possible. Aggregation should not be used to hide problems. Service level agreements should not be selected because the data are easily collected but because they are useful, for example, to identify and remedy process problems.

The customer and the vendor need to reach agreement on what will be measured and how. If the SLA involves availability, the period of time involved (a week, a month) should be stated. Will scheduled maintenance be excluded or included in calculating "uptime" for an application? For the user, loss of an application for any reason is "downtime," even if it is scheduled (Ferniany 2007).

From the user perspective, the inability to use an application makes it unavailable even if the problem is a broken hard drive or monitor. Vendors want to measure the availability of the application on the server or the availability of the network because they have the tools to measure that. There is no method for incorporating downtime related to desktop support or the help desk. The help desk and desktop support are treated as separate SLAs. For the physician or nurse, availability means being able to do their work. "What matters is what matters to the users," says Will Ferniany, PhD, chief executive officer of the University Hospitals and Clinics at the University of Mississippi Medical Center, who, until 2006, was senior vice president of administrative and network services at UPHS (see the case study at the end of part III).

Be careful about insisting on SLAs that use measures that are different from the ones used internally by the vendor. Take a look at what the vendor uses to measure quality, because it is more likely to measure those well. If the measures are acceptable, do not require different ones that the vendor may measure poorly or at greater cost. Remember that they are training staff and maintaining systems to create their internal measures (Ferniany 2007).

The objective set in the SLA should be affordable—that is, possible to achieve at a cost acceptable to the client (Sturm,

Morris, and Jander 2000, 67). While a client might desire that a system be available 99.999999 percent of the time, that level might not be possible at a cost the client is willing to pay, while 99.9 percent meets that test.

The SLA must represent something that is controllable. The "service provider must have the ability to exercise control over the factors that determine the level of service delivered" (Sturm, Morris, and Jander 2000, 65). Exclusions or waivers should be considered for factors that cannot be controlled. If the telephone company fails to honor a commitment to install phone lines to a building, the provider of IT services cannot be held accountable.

Both parties must agree to the SLA. Say the SLA states that 80 percent of total calls will be answered by a live agent within thirty seconds. The customer must understand the service, metric, and measurement. The understanding of the services provided should match the customer's expectations. Unrealistic or unreasonable expectations damage the client-provider relationship. While it may appear attractive for the customer to ask that 100 percent of total calls should be answered within 60 seconds, just one failure would mean that the provider had "failed" for that period. This may be an unreasonable expectation for IT, but it also offers no incentive for staff to comply for the rest of the reporting period.

Metrics

Table CS4-1 in the UPHS case study at the end of part III highlights sample service levels by major category and indicates what the service metric might be for each. For instance, under the category of Support Center/Help Desk, the individual SLA might be first-call resolution. The metric for this measure could be the number of calls resolved during the first contact with the help desk with a target measure such as 65 percent. Each individual SLA and its associated metric must be realistic, based on an organization's infrastructure.

Defining two levels of service may be desirable. The first is the minimum level of service that is considered acceptable, and a penalty could be defined for failure to reach that level. The second is the "stretch objective"—that is, a desired higher level of service (Sturm, Morris, and Jander 2000, 62). A third, "target" level might be the level of service that the provider expects to reach. The purpose of having multiple levels is to further define the expectations of both parties.

Having a stretch level in the SLA requires specifying a reward for the vendor for achieving that level. Possibilities include reducing a penalty for not achieving another SLA or making a bonus payment. The former undermines the concept of a minimum level of service. It would permit the vendor to reallocate resources without penalty. Bonus payments would require the establishment of a reserve fund for such payments. Health care organizations often lack sufficient funds for all the worthwhile projects they want to undertake—there are no unallocated funds. Senior managers will argue that a budget should be set for a desired level of service and improvements should be negotiated and budgeted in future years. Incentives are possible if the SLA can increase revenues or reduce costs. The incentives have to be self-funded. Ferniany (2007) says, "I can't give an incentive for making the network more reliable. There is no additional money there."

How Many Service Level Agreements Should We Have?

The number of metrics used will depend on the objectives of the customer and the provider. Using more SLAs increases the control of the customer. It can also provide opportunities for the provider to meet some of the SLAs and reduce the penalties for failure to deliver the primary service desired by the customer. For example, a lab might outsource the delivery of reports to an external vendor. What the lab wants is system availability 99.9 percent of the time so that lab reports can be transmitted. A single SLA could be written to hold the provider accountable. Alternatively, a series of SLAs could be negotiated that represent the components required to deliver that service, for example, SLAs for network availability, response time at the terminal ("screen flips"), and how quickly software upgrades are performed. Each SLA might have a penalty for missing the target. Now when the provider fails to meet the 99.9 percent availability target but meets several of the other SLAs, the penalties are less severe. Multiple SLAs might reduce the provider's incentive to deliver the ultimate service the customer wants.

Fewer SLAs, on the other hand, mean there is less to measure and, therefore, lower costs for the provider, which can be negotiated to mean lower costs for the customer. Fewer SLAs result in greater focus by both the customer and provider on the customer's ultimate objective. "Focus on a small number of SLAs. Extra SLAs require manpower to measure and monitor. Focus on the SLAs that explain most of the variance in performance" (Ferniany 2007).

> The number of metrics used will depend on the objectives of the customer and the provider. Using more SLAs increases the control of the customer. It can also provide opportunities for the provider to meet some of the SLAs and reduce the penalties for failure to deliver the primary service desired by the customer.

Customer Resistance

A radiology department that is negotiating an SLA with IT staff may resist an SLA with a level of service that is not ideal, for example, 24-hour-a-day, 365-day-a-year access to an image repository. Radiology may be unwilling to bear the cost of that level of availability or to reduce the level of availability. Negotiations can become contentious.

> Internal customers often resist the development of SLAs. It takes time to develop SLAs, and many internal customers do not want to spend that time. They are also concerned about being pinned down to a specific level of service, partly because they have never been asked to define the level of service they want nor confronted with the cost.

One solution may be to define SLAs iteratively over time. Both what is measured and the target level can be renegotiated after both parties experience a specific level of service. For example, the target for response to calls to a call center might be set at thirty seconds. After looking at the call abandonment rate, it may become clear that callers are willing to wait 40 seconds before a significant number of them abandon the call. The metric might be renegotiated to set a target for call abandonment instead of response time, or the target for response time might be renegotiated to a longer period that permits reduced staffing and lower cost.

Using Service Level Agreements Internally

While SLAs are often discussed as a tool for managing an outsourcing contract, they can be used in organizations that have chosen to continue to provide IT services with their own staff. Organizations have become more dependent on IT, and IT budgets have increased. Many CIOs are pressed to show that the millions invested in IT really benefit the organization. "To address these challenges, IT organizations should become service providers and structure their operations according to a service-provider model" (Garbani 2004, 2). Service level agreements are a part of what is called *service level management* (SLM). Service level agreements demonstrate a commitment to provide high-quality service to end users. The benefits of using SLAs internally include increased user satisfaction and productivity, increased consumer satisfaction, and increased IT staff productivity (Sturm, Morris, and Jander 2000, 126).

Service level agreements can be used for services other than IT. The University of Mississippi Medical Center (UMMC) is in the process of developing SLAs with support departments that are part of the University of Mississippi, which UMMC must use. Penalties are imposed for not meeting SLAs. Financial rewards are also offered for exceeding the SLAs. The University of Mississippi Medical Center's contracts with its practice plan groups in radiology, pathology, and radiation oncology provide for the sharing of technical fees if SLAs are met (Ferniany 2007).

In an outsourcing arrangement, the organization's CIO and some internal staff stay on the organization's payroll and continue to monitor operations. They understand the technology, so SLAs written in technical terms are understood. A challenge in developing SLAs for use internally is the very different perspectives and needs of IT providers and users. Users are concerned with whether they are able to do their work. Information technology is often "component centric," such that IT managers have historically measured the effectiveness of their organizations by looking at individual hardware and software components. Typically, the availability of components of a system is presented (e.g., network and servers), while from the user perspective the question is whether they could access all the resources needed to do their work. Sturm, Morris, and Jander (2000, 22) refer to this as "end to end" availability. For example, users might be concerned with the availability of an order entry system. Determining whether the application itself is running is not sufficient. The user is able to enter an order only when other components are available—for example, the network that links the user to the server on which the application runs. If availability to the user cannot be measured, then several measures must be used, returning to a component-centric point of view. The best approach may be to use both an end-to-end response time measure ("the time from when a command or transaction request is entered on the keyboard to the time when the resulting actions are completed and the results are displayed on the monitor" [Sturm, Morris, and Jander 2000, 1540) and a metric useful in diagnosing performance problems (e.g., the response time between servers involved in the transaction).

Even when IT creates a composite measure, it can be interpreted differently. So while IT may find system availability of 99.75 percent over a month acceptable, end users may be irate that there were 100 minutes during the month when they could not conduct business (Sturm, Morris, and Jander 2000, 11).

Another approach to categorizing SLAs reflects the ways users evaluate services rather than the components of the systems used. They are concerned about availability, performance, workload levels, security, accuracy, recoverability, and affordability (Sturm, Morris, and Jander 2000, 22). Performance, for example, could be measured by responsiveness to the request of a user (e.g., the repair or replacement of a computer) or the ability to meet a critical deadline. The SLAs written can include those needed by IT staff to diagnose problems and improve processes.

Sturm, Morris, and Jander (2000, 56) distinguish between in-house SLAs and internal SLAs. An *in-house* SLA is a formal agreement between a service provider and an in-house client (for examples, see the links to agreements at two schools of medicine in "Resources" at the end of this chapter). *Internal* SLAs are less formal; for example, they may be found in a number of documents—but they are written in technical terms nonetheless. They represent the expectations of the organization, including the CIO, for the performance of groups within the organization, for example, the network services group.

Even when an organization chooses to outsource its IT operations, some of the information presented to users should reflect their concerns and should be stated in terms they understand.

Role of Information Technology

The role of the IT department will be different, depending on the outsourcing relationship. Those differences must be understood in advance by the internal customers within the organization. When the outsourcing contract is signed with an external vendor, the role of IT is to manage the relationship with the vendor. If a unit of the organization has signed an agreement with an external vendor, the IT department's role may be as consultant to both the internal unit and the vendor. The IT department may also have an SLA with the unit. For example, a lab may have a contract with a vendor to provide reference services. It is the role of the lab, not the IT department, to manage its relationship with the reference service. The IT department might serve as a consultant, for example, advising the lab on how to negotiate an SLA that involves services delivered over the Internet. The IT department may also have an SLA with the lab to provide an internal network, for example, a wide area network that links all of the facilities in the organization.

Negotiating Service Level Agreements

Establishing SLAs between two parties is always challenging. Barriers exist that must be worked through in order to form a successful relationship. Current performance must be evaluated in order to establish new service levels, but this is often difficult to measure because of a lack of data. In addition, negotiating and defining SLAs is challenging because processes and tools often do not exist to enable measurement. These must be worked through and understood by both parties. Service level agreements can be difficult to measure, and organizational and process issues can sometimes impede an organization's ability to effectively measure. These process issues must also be addressed when establishing reasonable SLAs.

Service level agreements can be one sided. An organization may wish a vendor to achieve an SLA that is difficult to reach unless the organization makes investments it is unwilling or unable to make. The SLA may require that a network be available 99.9 percent of the time, but the age of the equipment used may make that extremely difficult to achieve. The vendor may try to negotiate a condition that hardware must be no more than three years old, but that investment may have a lower priority than others. In a competitive bidding process, a vendor may accept the SLA knowing it will be difficult to achieve. Both parties need to recognize the problem and work toward a resolution, which can be to ask the vendor to develop a plan for mitigating a problem while not imposing full penalties all the time. The organization can work to educate users and decision makers on the investment to maintain and improve services.

Three major considerations must be kept in mind during the negotiation (Garbani 2004, 6):

1. The benefits of a desired service level. It is necessary for the user of the service to understand the impact of a given service level and keep in mind the limits of the cost and performance trade-off parameters.

2. The cost of delivering a given service level. It is also necessary for the provider of the service to have a good understanding of the cost consequences of providing a specific level of service and to be able to justify the cost increase during the negotiation.

3. The availability of metrics. The provider of the service must be aware of its capabilities to accurately measure the service level using metrics. If, as is often the case, satisfactory data cannot be collected, the service provider must be prepared to explain what should be done and what cost will be incurred by adding a data collector.

If SLAs are used internally, then agreements should be reached one client at a time. "This ensures that the IT manager, acting in the role of service provider to various lines of business, can furnish the maximum attention to each client. It also guards against the confusion—and ultimately, the political upheaval and rebellion—that can erupt when multiple departments clamor at once to grasp new technology" (Sturm, Morris, and Jander 2000, 139).

Effect on Behavior

Service level agreements, if implemented correctly, can positively affect organizational behavior. For instance, they bring direct accountability by measuring performance and identifying areas for improvement. Service level agreements help end users by setting clear expectations and also presenting them with a reliable standard of service. End users can use SLAs to separate perception from reality when it comes to evaluating services performed. And finally, SLAs allow the IT department to "sell" a certain level of service to end users with confidence and be assured (within reason) of continuous improvement.

Service level agreements will direct where effort and resources go. They need to be selected carefully to prevent unwanted consequences. An SLA that requires help desk calls to be answered in thirty seconds or less could result in fewer problems being resolved during the first call. Help desk personnel may spend less time with callers and refer more of them to other staff. Requiring a higher percentage of problems to be resolved during the first call could result in longer calls and longer waits. Using both SLAs—for first-call resolution and answer time—could prevent this problem.

Too much of a focus on SLAs can cause resources to be concentrated on minimizing the negative in specific areas while ignoring improvement in others. A focus on quickly resolving user problems can take the place of efforts to educate users, for example.

Measuring Service Level Agreements

A number of steps can be taken to ensure that the effects of SLAs are measured accurately.

Establishing a Baseline

One of the most important components in developing appropriate SLAs is understanding current performance before establishing future measurement guidelines. If current performance is not analyzed, the target performance measures established might not be attainable. In addition, clarifying objectives and communicating them broadly are critical.

> Service level agreements are more than a tool for defining service. They create an infrastructure that supports true needs, solicits agreement of end users, serves as a tool to support higher budget requests, and is a foundation for a mutually advantageous relationship.

Service level agreements should not be a distraction. Only that which is meaningful should be measured so that administrative costs are reduced. Fewer SLAs should be in place, but they should carry higher rewards or penalties.

Measurement Tools

A strategy should be defined for capturing data and creating reports. Having the right tools in place to measure service levels is critical. When possible, automated tools should be used to measure automated processes. Such tools exist in many areas, including network performance, platform availability, and critical server uptime. For example, the uptime of critical servers can be measured by using server logs and continuous "ping" tests.[3]

For non-automated processes, people close to the situation (those who actually perform the processes) should be employed to measure them. These people will be the best educated on the SLAs, the processes being measured, and the SLAs' importance to their organization.

Cost of Service Level Agreements

The primary costs associated with implementing SLAs are (Sturm, Morris, and Jander 2000, 126):

- IT personnel to plan, implement, monitor, and report against service level agreements

---

[3] "(Packet INternet Groper) An Internet utility used to determine whether a particular [Internet Protocol (IP)] address is reachable online by sending out a packet and waiting for a response. Ping is used to test and debug a network as well as see if a user or server is online" (TechWeb 2006).

- Software costs for purchasing or developing tools to monitor, diagnose, manage, and report service quality, including problem notification
- Hardware costs for additional servers, workstations, and specialist equipment for supporting the service management software tools
- IT management attention to justify, procure software and hardware for, recruit and educate staff for, and oversee the operation of a service level management function

If SLAs are used in an outsourcing contract, the costs may not be visible to the client, but they still exist and are included in the cost of the agreement. However, large outsourcing organizations may incur lower costs because of existing licensing arrangements and the experience of their staff with these tools.

Software and hardware costs related to service level management will differ greatly according to the scale of the organization. A centralized IT organization that services multiple facilities will need more expensive tools than a single hospital. Software monitoring tools may be included in the purchase price of some hardware, for example, network routers. Organizations may need to acquire software reporting tools to merge and organize the data produced by existing hardware and software. Vendors should be consulted to determine if upgrades to existing software can provide reporting tools at a lower cost. The market for service level monitoring and reporting tools changes rapidly, so organizations will have to explore the options when they are ready (see the "Resources" section for SLAs following this chapter.)

Real-time data are needed by providers in order to avoid paying penalties. If an SLA requires that the provider meet a target each month, current status is needed to allow time for corrective action.

Resources

Time and Motion Studies

Agency for Healthcare Research and Quality, "Using Time and Motion Studies to Measure the Impact of Health IT on Clinical Workflow": "Researchers at Partners Healthcare have created a tool to help others accurately capture time and motion study data. The tool—a Microsoft Access database—allows observers to record time and motion data and store them for analysis. In addition, Partners has created a user's guide for this new tool and published a journal article that provides a case example of how the tool can be used to evaluate the effectiveness of a health information technology. Together, the tool, the user's guide, and the journal article can help you measure the impact of technology on clinical workflow." Available for download at http://healthit.ahrq.gov. Enter "EHR Time & Motion Tool" in the Search box.

Service Level Agreements

"IT Infrastructure Library" guidelines have been developed by the Office of Governance Commerce (www.itil.org/en/index.php) in Norwich, England, for the British government. It is considered by some to be the principal standard for service management.

Links to service level management software compiled by Bitpipe, Inc. (http://www.bitpipe.com/olist/Service-Level-Management.html).

nextslm.org is a Web site on service level management sponsored by BMC Software (www.nextslm.org).

slminfo.org is a Web site on service level management sponsored by Enterprise Management Associates (http://www.slminfo.com).

The IT Services Service Level Agreement (including individual SLAs) was developed by Information Technology Services at the University of Washington School of Medicine (http://home.mcis.washington.edu/amcis/services/).

A template used in writing a service level agreement for data center services was developed by Information Technology Services at the Stanford University School of Medicine and is available online (http://med.stanford.edu/irt/datacenter/sla.html). This is the template for a contract, but it includes SLAs.

References
for Chapters 7–9

Badger, Stephen, Ryan Bosch, and Praveen Toteja. 2005. Rapid implementation of an electronic health record in an academic setting. *Journal of Healthcare Information Management* 19 (2): 34–40.

Carr, Jim. 2001. Service level agreements. June 5. http://www. networkcomputing.com/showArticle/.jhtml?articleID=8703118 (accessed May 8, 2007).

Domalewski, Mark, and Patricia Berger. 2005. PACS—Is it a measurable success? Paper presented at the Healthcare Information and Management Systems Society Conference and Exhibition, Dallas, TX, February 15, 2005.

Ferniany, Will, PhD, CEO, University Hospitals and Clinics, The University of Mississippi Medical Center. 2007. Personal communication.

Garbani, Jean-Pierre. 2004. *Best practices for service level management.* Cambridge, MA: Forrester.

Levinson, Meridith. 2003. It ain't over until you do the post-implementation audit. *CIO Magazine,* October 1. http://www.cio.com/au/index.php/id;1091307774 (accessed May 8, 2007).

Massachusetts Technology Collaborative and New England Healthcare Institute. 2006. Computerized physician order entry. Lessons learned from community hospitals. November. http://www.fcg.com/research/research-listing.aspx?rid=318&NoIntro=True (accessed February 5, 2007).

Mekhjian, Hagop, Rajee Kumar, Lynn Kuehn, et. al. 2002. Immediate benefits realized following implementation of physician order entry at an academic medical center. *Journal of the American Medical Informatics Association* 9 (6): 529–39. http://www.jamia.org/cgi/content/full/9/5/529 (accessed May 8, 2007).

Murphy, Tony. 2002. *Achieving business value from technology: A practical guide for today's executive.* Hoboken, NJ: John Wiley & Sons.

Pizziferri, Lisa, Anne Kittler, Lynn Volk, et. al. 2005. Primary care physician time utilization before and after implementation of an electronic health record: A time-motion study. *Journal of Biomedical Informatics* 38 (3): 176–88. www.sciencedirect.com (accessed November 21, 2006).

Sturm, Rick, Wayne Morris, and Mary Jander. 2000. *Foundations of service level management.* Indianapolis, IN: Sams.

Taylor, Rick, John Manzo, and Mark Sinnett. 2002. Quantifying value for physician order-entry systems: A balance of cost and quality. *Healthcare Financial Management* 56 (7): 44–48.

TechWeb. 2006. TechEncylopedia. http://www.techweb.com/encyclopedia/ (accessed September 14, 2006).

Thompson, Douglas, Sharon Henry, Linda Lockwood, Brian Anderson, and Susan Atkinson. 2005. Benefits planning for advanced clinical information systems implementation at Allina Hospitals and Clinics. *Journal of Healthcare Information Management* 19 (1): 54–62.

Case Study No. 3

Banner Estrella Medical Center: Determining the Benefits of Care Transformation and Information Technology Implementation

Banner Estrella Medical Center (BEMC) in Phoenix, Arizona, is a 172-bed hospital that opened in February 2005. It is a new hospital in a new location, not a replacement facility. Banner Estrella Medical Center is owned by Banner Health, a not-for-profit health care system. Banner Health's leadership decided to use the planning and design of BEMC as a "conduit to transform how we deliver care throughout the organization. We would use the rollout of HIT as a way to fundamentally examine and revamp how Banner delivers care at every hospital, looking for best practices and standardization" (Warden and Van Norman 2006). Banner Health functions as a single operating company rather than a holding company for hospitals operating under their own principles, operating structure, and support systems. The health system began to plan a new care transformation design, with technology at the core. Implementation at each location would be completed by December 31, 2008.

Judy Van Norman, system director of care transformation at Banner Health, says, "Banner Estrella is our prototype and test bed. Now, when I talk with the other hospitals, I don't have to ask them to take my word for anything. I say: The benefits are real—go see them. Go talk to your counterpart at Estrella. Care transformation is not just a concept anymore" (Intel 2007).

The care transformation effort is a multiyear plan that will cost more than $100 million for the entire Banner Health system. It utilizes enabling technology such as electronic medical records, automated alerts, and CPOE to transform patient care into safe processes that can be executed with little variation. The principal software is Cerner Millennium®, a product of the Cerner Corporation, which provides software to the health care industry (www.cerner.com).

Banner Health

Based in Phoenix, Banner Health has twenty facilities that offers an array of services, including hospital care, home care, hospice care, nursing registries, surgery centers, laboratories, and rehabilitation services. These facilities are located in seven states—Alaska, Arizona, California, Colorado, Nebraska, Nevada, and Wyoming. Banner has 3,065 licensed acute hospitals beds, employs more than 25,000 employees, and has $3 billion in annual revenue (Banner Health 2006).

Banner Health was created in 1999 by the merger of the former Samaritan Health System of Phoenix and the Lutheran Health System of Fargo, North Dakota. Its hospitals range in size from 600-bed Banner Good Samaritan Hospital in Phoenix to thirty-bed facilities in Wyoming and Nebraska.

Care Transformation

The care transformation initiative is the combination of technology, process redesign, evidence-based best practices, and the cultural transformation necessary to make the adoption successful. Banner Health involved 300 clinicians from across the organization in identifying and standardizing best practices. Once determined, Banner used culture change, workflow redesign, and technology to implement them at BEMC.

Each hospital employs a care transformation deployment manager, all of whom are nurses. They serve as the project manager for care transformation at their hospital. Half of their time is spent at the corporate level, and the other half is spent coordinating and managing the rollout of care transformation at their hospital. Work redesign is supported by a group of management engineers.[1] Each hospital maintains a deployment council, made up of department managers and executives. "The council operates as the facility's care transformation sponsor, charged with training, communication, and ultimately encouraging acceptance of the new methods and standardization" (Warden and Van Norman 2006).

"Making a success out of Banner Estrella was vital. Other Banner hospitals would see what success looked like there, and quickly be able to make the connection about the importance and necessity of care transformation. While it is easy to naysay something in the concept stage, it is much more difficult to turn down a proven product or method. It is nearly impossible to say or to believe something doesn't work when, in fact, it does work" (Warden and Van Norman 2006).

Objectives for the redesign include (Warden and Van Norman 2006):

- Fewer handoffs and work queues
- Intuitive system development to promote ease of use
- One set of screen formats and data definitions
- One set of consistent core reports across facilities
- Standard system outputs across facilities

To revamp Banner's care, the team, assembled from across the system, redesigned 92 processes in 11 key areas (Warden and Van Norman 2006):

- Care management
- Clinical documentation
- CPOE
- Document imaging
- Emergency services

---

[1]*Management engineering* is the name commonly given to the industrial engineering discipline when it is applied within health care settings (Health Information and Management Systems Society 2007).

- Medication administration
- Obstetrics
- Orders management/nursing orders
- Pediatrics
- Scheduling
- Surgery

Information Technology and Care Transformation

Banner Health had already been using IT to improve clinical practice. A group began working in 1994 at Good Samaritan Regional Medical Center to develop a method of reducing injury from adverse drug events[2] using the decision support capability of Cerner's Discern Expert information system (Raschke et al. 1998).

The IT implemented at BEMC included an inpatient and emergency department EMR, CPOE, decision support software, and PACS.

Banner Health wanted to implement real-time decision support for clinicians. In the two years preceding BEMC's opening, Banner clinicians and informaticists[3] analyzed work flow and mapped Banner's needs to the capabilities of Cerner Millennium and other IT applications. Nurses configured their portion of the EMR, and physicians reached consensus on evidence-based order sets.

To develop the order sets, Banner convened a physician advisory council. The group, composed of a representative from every medical specialty offered, created approximately 120 cross-team order sets for BEMC's launch. The order sets included a wide variety of common diagnoses and procedures.

---

[2]"Adverse Drug Event (ADE)—An adverse event involving medication use. Examples: anaphylaxis to penicillin, major hemorrhage from heparin, aminoglycoside-induced renal failure, agranulocytosis from chloramphenicol" (Agency for Healthcare Research and Quality 2007).

[3]An *informaticist* applies information technology to a specific discipline.

"What quickly became apparent was the need to consolidate around specific drugs, specific doses and balancing order sets so that the vast majority of what a physician would need would be readily available. The valuable input from the council meant the care transformation team would begin from the start with guidelines championed by our physicians" (Warden and Van Norman 2006).

The care transformation team created a system in which data elements, documentation, and applications were built and standardized with naming conventions, forms, flow sheets, and screen formats for all Banner hospitals. While physicians can utilize the order sets, they are not mandatory. The order sets are intended to expedite the ordering process.

Banner Estrella has a new medical staff. Some physicians applied for medical staff membership, while others were recruited. The medical staff bylaws for BEMC were intentionally written to require that physicians use CPOE and receive system training. Physicians who utilize CPOE for less than 85 percent of their orders are asked to have a discussion with the chief medical officer (CMO). "Rather than forcing them to sign off on it before their first day, however, we spent countless hours working for physicians' approval and belief in the care transformation vision" (Warden and Van Norman 2006).

Charlie Agee, MD, CMO of Banner Estrella Medical Center, reports that "within six months of opening, we could have had physicians try to derail it. We tried to get physician champions to buy in. It was taking them more time, but we asked them to wait and see the benefits. More and more people bought into it. They have to be willing to spend the time to learn how to use the system."

Benefits Determination

Together, staff from Banner Health, Cerner, and Intel examined data relating to key performance indicators for the operational period of January through June 2006, the most recent period for which data were available. They used the Intel Healthcare IT Economic Model (www.intel.com/healthcare/healthit).

The benefits study will be used to sustain the momentum as care transformation is rolled out across the other facilities. The study fulfills a promise to the board of directors to conduct an analysis of the benefits received. Those who are oriented to the bottom line also want to know what effect care transformation is having. Those who believe there are better department-specific IT solutions need to be convinced of the benefits of an integrated IT architecture. System Director Van Norman emphasizes, "Monetizing benefits is important because money is a common language, but the real reason we're doing this is to improve patient care."

Banner Health needs to know if this model is working before it is replicated for all its hospitals. Improvements can also be made in the systems operating at BEMC. New features are piloted at BEMC before they are rolled out to other facilities.

Because they could not do "before and after" analysis of a new hospital, the team compared BEMC to a "virtual hospital" based on the weighted average of eight Banner Health hospitals that had not fully implemented care transformation. The eight Banner hospitals were selected because they were of similar bed size as BEMC or larger. A heart hospital was excluded because of the differences in services provided. Six of the eight hospitals were already using Cerner Millennium in 2005, but none had implemented CPOE.

The team looked at ten key indicators and identified up to $2.8 million in financial benefits for the six-month period by calculating the difference between BEMC and the virtual hospital. The result showed (Intel 2007):

- Lower average length of stay (ALOS)
- Lower overtime expenditure per 1,000 admissions
- Lower drug expenditure per 1,000 adjusted admissions (adjusted for case mix)
- Lower form expenditure per 1,000 admissions

- Lower document storage costs per 1,000 admissions
- Greater avoidance of costs for treating adverse drug events per 1,000 acute admissions
- Fewer medication-related malpractice insurance claims per 1,000 acute admissions
- Fewer days in accounts receivable (AR)
- Fewer nurses leaving voluntarily within the first year of employment
- More emergency department (ED) visitors treated (because fewer patients left without treatment)

The greatest bottom-line impact resulted from improvements in ALOS, a drop in the number of patients who left the ED without treatment, pharmacy cost reduction, and ADE avoidance (figure CS3-1). Average length of stay, adjusted for case mix, was 7 percent lower than at the virtual hospital, and pharmacy costs, also case-mix adjusted, were 18 percent lower.

The financial effect of ALOS reduction was measured by the variable cost per day avoided. Adverse drug event avoidance was measured by determining the number of alerts sent, or "fired," by the system and the number of changes that were subsequently made to orders. Banner Health had been using this technology since the 1990s (Raschke et al. 1998). The benefit is the incremental improvement in how often a physician changes an order after an alert. Compared to facilities that had front-end pharmacy alerts in place but did not have CPOE, BEMC had 84 percent more therapy changes per 1,000 acute admissions, helping BEMC avoid the cost and resources (and its patients avoid the time and pain) of treating potential complications. The dollar value of an avoided ADE is assumed to be $4,000, based on prior studies done elsewhere.[4]

---

[4]Including a study by Bates, Spell, and Cullen (1997): "The additional length of stay associated with an ADE was 2.2 days (P = .04), and the increase in cost associated with an ADE was $3244 (P = .04). For preventable ADEs, the increases were 4.6 days in length of stay (P = .03) and $5857 in total cost (P = .07). After adjusting for our sampling strategy, the estimated postevent costs attributable to an ADE were $2595 for all ADEs and $4685 for preventable ADEs."

Figure CS3-1.   Banner Estrella Medical Center Final Set of Findings

Economic Effect	Total Effect w/o CM	Bottom Line Change w/o CM	Total Effect w/CM	Bottom Line Change w/CM	Just AZ Bottom Line w/CM
ALOS Reduction	$ 4,340,696	$1,781,544	$1,324,067	$ 543,434	$ 666,167
Overtime Reduction	$ 74,652	$ 30,639	$ 74,652	$ 30,639	$ (6,990)
Pharmacy Cost Reduction	$ 785,478	$ 322,382	$ 318,615	$ 130,769	$ 109,940
Form Elimination	$ 54,526	$ 22,379	$ 54,526	$ 22,379	$ 18,931
Document Storage Cost Reduction	$ 26,711	$ 26,711	$ 26,711	$ 26,711	$ 26,711
ADE Avoidance	$ 290,134	$ 119,079	$ 290,134	$ 119,079	$ 119,368
Med-related claims avoidance	$ 89,308	$ 89,308	$ 64,118	$ 64,118	$ 80,704
Days in AR Reduction	$ 18,416	$ 18,416	$ 18,416	$ 18,416	$ 18,416
Nurse Retention	$ 37,576	$ 37,576	$ 37,576	$ 37,576	$ 37,576
Fewer ED LWOTs	$ 339,766	$ 339,766	$ 339,766	$ 339,766	$ 584,284
Total with ALOS (6 mos)	$ 6,057,262	$2,787,801	$2,548,581	$1,332,888	$1,655,107
Total without ALOS (6 mos)	$ 1,716,566	$1,006,257	$1,224,514	$ 789,453	$ 988,940
Total with ALOS (Annualized)	$12,114,524	$5,575,602	$5,097,161	$2,665,775	$3,310,214
Total without ALOS (Annualized)	$ 3,433,132	$2,012,513	$2,449,027	$1,578,907	$1,977,881

Note: ADE = adverse drug event; ALOS = average length of stay; AR = accounts receivable; AZ = Arizona; CM = case-mix adjustment; ED LWOT = emergency department visitors leaving without treatment.

Source: Reprinted with permission of Banner Health.

Other benefits contributing to the $2.8 million in financial benefits for the six-month period were:

- Overtime expense was 5 percent lower.
- Forms costs were more than 40 percent less.
- Bills spent a day less in AR, allowing quicker payment.
- Retention of nurses in their first year of Banner employment was higher, reducing hiring and training costs.
- The cost of medication-related malpractice insurance claims per 1,000 acute admissions (adjusted for case mix) was 72 percent lower.

Some effects of changes could not be measured because of the limitations of existing data. For example, the time accounting system does not allow for the determination of nurse overtime related to documentation. While interview data suggested that the new systems were shortening documentation time, that specific effect could not be accurately measured.

Bottom-Line Impact

The $2.8 million included only savings that would have an effect on the bottom line, defined as earnings before interest, taxes, depreciation, and amortization (EBITDA). With the exception of additional revenue in the ED, the benefits were achieved by avoiding costs (e.g., overtime and document storage).

The type of payment for an episode of care affects whether or not a hospital financially benefits from a change. For example, shortening the length of stay of a Medicare patient would reduce the hospital's costs but not decrease revenue, because payment is made on an all-inclusive case rate based on diagnosis-related group (DRG). Shortening the length of stay when the hospital is paid a per-diem rate would lower both costs and revenues. To adjust for the type of payment, a bottom-line change was calculated for each benefit (figure CS3-1).

Per-diem reimbursement is approximately 59 percent of BEMC's revenue. The remaining 41 percent of revenue is per-case payment or capitation. Only 41 percent of the total savings from items related to ALOS was, therefore, included in the bottom-line change (figure CS3-1). Savings from document storage cost reduction, medication-related claims avoidance, days in AR reduction, nurse retention, and fewer instances of patients leaving the ED without treatment were considered to be unaffected by length of stay and were not adjusted.

Case-Mix Adjustment

Banner Estrella Medical Center is a new facility that does not have some services, including specialized pediatrics. It is also a Level II, not a Level I, trauma center. The demographics of the community include both a large elderly population and a significant number of births because of the number of young families moving into the hospital's service area in the West Valley, a growing area of Phoenix. Differences in the case mix of patients at BEMC and the virtual hospital could partially explain the differences in costs. Case-mix adjustment was used to attempt to compensate for differences in the types of patients seen. Figure CS3-1 shows values with and without case-mix adjustment.

Some effects are assumed to be sensitive to differences in case mix, including ALOS reduction, pharmacy cost reduction, and medication-related claims reduction. An adjustment was made to account for differences in the case mix at BEMC and the eight hospitals used to create a virtual hospital. Case-mix index (CMI) adjustment was done for medication-related claims reduction with the assumption that more severe cases result in higher liability claims.

For pharmacy cost reduction and medication-related cost reduction, the following case-mix adjustment method was used. The data for BEMC were divided by its CMI. The data for each of the eight hospitals were also divided by its CMI. A weighted average of the results for the eight hospitals was calculated using admissions (i.e., data for each hospital were multiplied by the percentage of total admissions for the eight hospitals at that hospital). For ALOS reduction, case-mix adjustment was done

DRG by DRG. The ALOS for each diagnosis-related group at BEMC was determined. This was compared to the ALOS at each of the other eight hospitals.

Adjusting for case mix and considering only bottom-line impact, the benefits were estimated to be $1.3 million for a six-month period, or $2.7 million annually. The total savings without ALOS reduction is presented in figure CS3-1. Excluding ALOS reduction lowers the savings. (Banner Health sought a high and low estimate of benefits.) Results are also shown when the comparison is restricted to only Arizona hospitals, which results in a higher benefits estimate (figure CS3-1). (Because of the regulatory and pricing environment specific to Arizona, Banner sought a separate estimate using data only for Arizona hospitals to create the virtual hospital.)

Extrapolating to Other Facilities

The benefits study was undertaken to estimate the benefits from care transformation at BEMC. Other Banner facilities may see higher or lower benefits. A major risk in extrapolating the results at BEMC to other Banner hospitals is whether physicians will utilize CPOE, a requirement for getting medical staff membership at BEMC. Transitioning away from the paper chart may also have to happen incrementally because of the comfort level of staff with using paper. The benefits may be achieved more slowly. Van Norman notes that "implementing care transformation at existing hospitals is like rewiring cars when they are running."

The larger volume of patients at other Banner hospitals will result in higher total dollar benefits. Banner Estrella also has a higher proportion of per-diem payment. Hospitals with a higher proportion of per-case payment (e.g., a larger Medicare population) would see greater bottom-line savings.

Why Are Benefits Received?

Banner Health is attempting to transform how care is provided. Information technology has enabled the changes to varying degrees. No attempt has been made to separate the effect of changes in how care is provided (e.g., changes in work flow, use of order sets) from functions available through IT (e.g., automated alerts, decision support for ordering). Nor has any attempt been made to isolate the effects of BEMC's innovative architecture and services (Banner Health 2006; McGuigan 2006).

Some benefits are easy to explain. Bills spent a day less in AR, allowing quicker payment. Because the medical record is online, the medical coders in billing do not have to wait until a paper record reaches them to start their work.

To understand what changes were occurring, interviews were conducted to understand how staff, including physicians and nurses, viewed the changes. Interviews also identified multi-disciplinary work flow benefits. The interviews focused on the work flow for that person. The interviews revealed other data that should be acquired to augment the initial data request. The results suggest the reasons that the benefits were received. Some of the results are organized below by type of benefit.

Average Length of Stay Reduction

Physicians say the tools help them do a better job for their patients. Chief Medical Officer Dr. Agee says, "Your brain can remember most things most of the time. When you have a system, that system prompts you for the correct medications, doses and frequencies, it takes care of a lot of the rote memory work. It frees up brain cells so you can use your clinical acumen more creatively to optimize the care of this particular patient" (Intel 2007).

Banner Estrella Medical Center clinicians say the IT-rich BEMC environment and the cross-enterprise care transformation process foster a more holistic, team-oriented approach to patient care—one they believe improves outcomes and enhances job satisfaction. According to John Placko, RPh, director of pharmacy at BEMC, "Physicians, nurses and ancillary services at Banner Estrella are more tightly integrated. We all have a better understanding of how we impact each other. It is a whole different mind set, and very beneficial for the patient" (Intel 2007).

Clinicians collaborate more effectively in real time. Agee notes, "In the paper world, there is *one* chart. With the EMR, we can have a hospitalist, a radiologist, and a consultant all looking at the chart at the same time, to improve on outcomes in a quicker fashion. You can also sit down with the patient, use a tablet or a computer on wheels to show them their radiological studies in real time, and make decisions together right at the bedside." Everyone from respiratory therapists to dietitians can engage with the patient sooner and be a better informed partner in patient care (Intel 2007).

Adverse Drug Events and Pharmacy Cost Reduction

Joel McAlduff, MD, system director for medical informatics and clinical innovation at Banner Health, says, "Orders are dispatched with more immediacy because of the technologies. They're more likely to be the right orders because physicians are following evidence-based order sets, and they're alerted to any incompatibilities or allergies. Test results come back faster because we've removed the delays that are inherent in a paper system. Handwriting errors and unapproved abbreviations—both big sources of error—are eliminated. And when treatment guidelines change, we can embed [the changes] into the system and change our practices quickly" (Intel 2007).

Pharmacists do not have to scratch their heads trying to figure out what the doctor has written. Director of Pharmacy Placko says, "They're free to focus on what is going on with the patient and the appropriateness of the therapy. That reduces errors and generates savings in the long run, and enables pharmacists to make a more valuable contribution." Pharmacy costs have also been affected by process changes and by the standardization of care sets, among other factors. According to Placko, "Care sets help reduce inventory costs because we've reduced the number of items we need to order" (Intel 2007).

Data on orders and alerts can be used to avoid ADEs. The Food and Drug Administration (FDA) had recently placed an alert on the use of the drug promethazine in patients under the age of two, due to respiratory depression. Banner Health pharmacists were not overly concerned, as they were under the impression that the medication was rarely used by physicians for this age group. A quick search of the Cerner Millennium database at BEMC and at another Banner hospital, however, revealed seven uses of the drug. Within hours, a rule was written alerting physicians to the FDA's warning on promethazine orders for patients under the age of two. Days later, an audit of that specific alert determined the rule "fired" (appeared to the physician on the screen) six times, and in all six cases the physician cancelled the order. This is an example of what Van Norman calls "hardwiring." The change does not rely on the memory of clinicians or the actions of administrative and clerical staff.

"Without this technology, Banner could not have disseminated the alert so quickly, or known if it was acted upon. Physicians can immediately make a change where appropriate, before the initial order transaction occurs, whereas in non-CPOE facilities, a pharmacist would have to track down the ordering physician to relay the information" (Warden and Van Norman 2006).

Nurse Retention and Overtime Reduction

Nurses see care transformation as a tremendous resource to make them better, more efficient nurses. Diane Drexler, RN, chief nursing officer at BEMC, says, "Because of the EMR, nurses have the whole picture. They can develop a better plan of care and intervene more effectively for their patients because they've got all the information at their fingertips. When a patient is admitted from the Emergency Department, the floor nurses are better prepared for them because they can see the information that [has] already been collected. They can utilize resources more effectively and move the patient along in their recovery more quickly. If they call a physician, they're not scrambling to find the chart when the physician calls back" (Intel 2007).

Nurses also say they can manage their time more effectively, which relieves stress and enhances care. Debbie Carter, RN, deployment manager at BEMC, adds, "Nurses have time to develop more empathy with the patient. They can listen more closely without feeling stressed out because they're not getting their charting done. It's a wonderful feeling" (Intel 2007).

Lessons Learned

Van Norman believes that "it is important to do a benefit study to support the case for large investments like an EMR, even when we intuitively feel it is the right thing to do. However, it is difficult to determine the cause of the benefits when there are so many other changes going on as we try to improve quality and patient safety. It is important to have the anecdotal data to give you confidence that you are looking in the right places for the benefits. If clinicians tell you that the system is not creating a collaborative environment and that they hated using it, you'd have to look at the measured benefits with skepticism."

References

Agency for Healthcare Research and Quality. 2007. Patient safety network: Glossary. www.psnet.ahrq.gov/glossary.aspx (accessed February 14, 2007).

Banner Health. 2006. Banner Estrella programs and services. www.bannerhealth.com/Locations/Arizona/Banner+Estrella+Medical+Center/Programs+and+Services/_Programs+and+Services.htm (accessed January 18, 2007).

Bates, D., N. Spell, and D. Cullen. 1997. The costs of adverse drug events in hospitalized patients. Adverse Drug Events Prevention Study Group. *Journal of the American Medical Association* 277 (4): 307–11.

Health Information and Management Systems Society. 2007. What is a management engineer or process improvement professional? www.himss.org/asp/topics_FocusDynamic.asp?faid=105 (accessed February 14, 2007).

Intel. 2007. *Intel case study: Healing environment, proven value*. Santa Clara, CA: Intel.

McGuigan, C. 2006. Design for a healing space. *Newsweek,* October 16. www.msnbc.msn.com/id/15175919/site/newsweek/page/10 (accessed January 18, 2007).

Raschke, R., B. Gollihare, T. Wunderlich, et. al. 1998. A computer alert system to prevent injury from adverse drug events. *Journal of the American Medical Association* 280 (15): 1317–20.

Warden, M., and J. Van Norman. 2006. Franchising for the future of care. Cerner Quarterly, www.cerner.com/public/*CernerQuarterly.* asp?id=28348 (accessed January 17, 2007).

Case Study No. 4

University of Pennsylvania Health System: Development and Use of Service Level Agreements

IN JANUARY 2001, the University of Pennsylvania Health System (UPHS) announced the signing of a five-year agreement with First Consulting Group (FCG) (www.fcg.com) and Affiliated Computer Services (ACS) (www.acs-inc.com) for the provision to UPHS of specialized health care information technology management services. This outsourcing agreement was "expected to save UPHS approximately $19 million in operating costs over the life of the contract. Under the terms of the agreement, FCG and ACS (operating as a subcontractor to FCG and providing services through its operating division, ACS Health Solutions) will operate as a team with current UPHS information services leadership to manage the Health System[']s information systems infrastructure and applications support" (UPHS 2001). The agreement was extended for one additional year in March 2006.

Under the terms of the agreement, with an estimated value of $100 million, FCG assumed direct responsibility for managing a variety of UPHS IT functions, including its help desk, local area networks, applications support, and applications upgrades. Affiliated Computer Services would manage mainframe and mid-range computer operations and wide area networking and would join FCG in service level management. University of Pennsylvania Health System would retain most of the IT responsibility for its School of Medicine and telecommunications divisions as well as its Phoenixville Hospital facility (UPHS 2001).

Included in the contract were service level agreements (SLAs) that defined the minimum levels of performance in areas such as network availability and help desk performance (table CS4-1). This case describes the experience of UPHS in using SLAs from 2001 to 2006.

University of Pennsylvania Health System

University of Pennsylvania Health System (http://pennhealth.com) is a multihospital system with headquarters in Philadelphia. It includes three wholly owned hospitals: Hospital of the University of Pennsylvania, Pennsylvania Hospital, and Penn Presbyterian Medical Center. University of Pennsylvania Health System also includes the University of Pennsylvania School of Medicine, educationally affiliated hospitals, multispecialty satellite facilities, a primary care provider network, home health care, and hospice and long-term care.

Value of Service Level Agreements

George Brenckle, PhD, UPHS's CIO, believes that SLAs have "turned out to be an incredibly valuable management tool that gives you and your customers insight on what is happening in the organization and some transparency to what is happening. They help you have a dialogue about expectations. They provide insight about what worked, what the issues were and where the work was."

University of Pennsylvania Health System outsourced in 2001, but it took six months to decide on the SLAs that went into the request for proposals (RFPs). Originally, 400 SLAs were enumerated in the contract, but Brenckle quickly realized he needed to pay close attention to about 40 to 50 of them and that he rarely looked at 300 of them. First Consulting Group requested changes to about 50 of them, but they have remained in the contract.

The health system's contract with FCG and ACS expires in March 2007. After five years, it is now easy to make clear to vendors exactly what UPHS expects and what the history has been. In the RFP for the new contract, vendors have been given historical data for the SLA metrics so that they can see what

Table CS4-1. Selected University of Pennsylvania Health System Service Level Agreements

Standard SLA Samples			Sample SLA Standards & Metrics	
Service	Item	Individual SLA	Metric %	Service Metric
Support Center/Help Desk	1	Help Desk First Call Resolution	65.00%	Resolution of calls @ first contact that are within the scope of help desk staff resolution
	2	Answer Time	80.00%	Answered within 30 seconds
	3	Abandoned Call	≤5%	Maximum calls abandoned over 20 seconds
	5	User Satisfaction Survey—Help Desk	80.00%	Minimum monthly average survey score
Data Center Services	6	Data Backup	99.00%	Backups completed within scheduled time
	7	Data Restore	100.00%	Successful restores completed within scheduled time
	8	Server Availability	Mission Critical 99.5% Non Mission Critical 98.5%	Total measure of scheduled and unscheduled availability, servers % mission critical servers and non-mission critical servers respectively
	9	Disaster Recovery Testing	100.00%	100% of scheduled activities completed and 100% tested and re-tested activities
Network Services	10	Network Performance	99.00%	Network backbone availability
	11	Equipment/Software Release Mgmt.	99.00%	Installs completed as scheduled
Desktop Services	12	Break/Fix Resolution	98.00%	Successful resolution of break/fix tickets within 1 business day
	13	Moves/Adds/Changes Performed	99.00%	Successful completion within 10 business days

Source: Reprinted with permission of University of Pennsylvania Health System.

work has taken place. This time, it has taken one month instead of six months to write the RFP.

Bill Weber, FCG's account manager at UPHS, believes that SLAs define the minimum level of service to be provided to the end user. "You can't have a good contract without that. If we don't have that, the services I needed to provide would be a moving target. In most cases they are not, by any means, the level you want to strive for." Service level agreements provide the vendor with the opportunity to make some decisions about where resources will be used to either meet or exceed the SLA. Some SLAs do represent targets to strive for, for example, 99.9 percent network availability.

Weber hopes that SLAs will develop into a method for setting mutual expectations and be less one sided. For example, an SLA for network availability would require that a vendor ensure that a network is operating 99.99 percent of the time, but the client would agree in the contract that the equipment is no more than three years old. Weber believes there is a tendency now to say that because the vendor has agreed to the SLA, the client does not need to make changes. However, both parties are interested in providing a high level of service.

Developing Service Level Agreements

Brenckle cautions that organizations need to be careful in selecting measures, because they will direct where effort and resources go. If a service level is set requiring help desk calls to be answered in thirty seconds or less, then calls will be short and perhaps will not solve the problem. If a service level is set that stipulates the percentage of problems that must be resolved on the first call, then the length of calls will increase and the time before calls are answered will increase. An SLA can make a situation worse. How people will react may not be known in advance. One of the advantages of starting with a larger number of SLAs and then reducing them is that you avoid having the focus shift to just one element of a service. "You realize that although you have eight to nine service levels, here are the four that help me optimize. The rest are my supports," says Brenckle.

The SLAs include measures of end user satisfaction. Brenckle believes that averages do not work. "If there's a scale of 1–5, the percent of people who respond with the poorest score, a one, may better reflect the general feeling about a service. It reflects the small group of people who are very dissatisfied." Weber agrees. When the percentage of people who rate a service negatively during a week goes above 2 percent, it is accompanied by verbal complaints and negative e-mails. Figure CS4-1 shows the percentage of responses where satisfaction was rated the lowest—that is, a 1. Figure CS4-2 shows the number of such responses. While the trend in both metrics is generally downward, there is considerable variability month to month.

Besides customer satisfaction, measures of productivity are important. With flat expenditures for IT but a growing number of clinical applications, getting more from the same resources has become important. Brenckle believes that better measures are needed for applications development and maintenance services (ADMS). Programmer and interface developer productivity is hard to measure when the work is on purchased software. "You struggle to measure output, so you measure input," according to Brenckle.

Further, he says,

> The issue is that the other IT services are more standard in nature and easier to count. In ADMS, a "change to an interface" could be a 4 hour effort or it could be a 4 week effort. It is not easy to have an objective sense of the right amount of effort for a given task. If an enhancement is budgeted for 8 hours and takes 16 hours—is that because the estimate was wrong or because the person doing the work was not efficient? Do you set a service level for meeting estimates? Wouldn't that motivate people to estimate high? In short, ADMS suffers from the large degree of variability in the tasks. Some people swear by "function points," which may work in a true software development environment [Herron 2000]. But in an environment where you are supporting package applications, function points are not easy to adapt.

Figure CS4-1. University of Pennsylvania Health System Negative (1) Survey Response Percentage

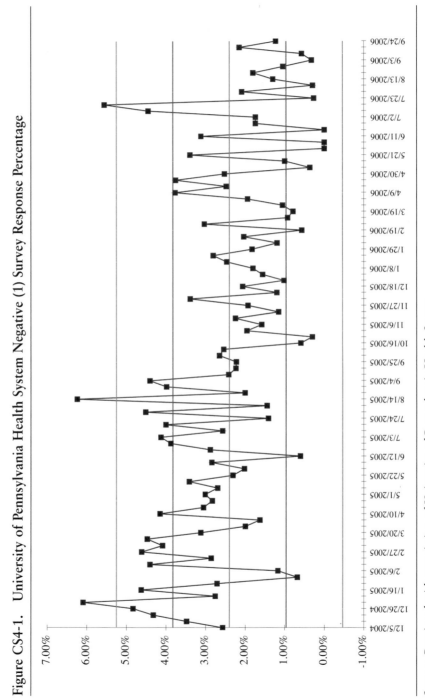

Source: Reprinted with permission of University of Pennsylvania Health System.

226

Figure CS4-2. Information Services Survey Count of 1s

227

Service level agreements require customers to define their expectations—what will make them happy. Brenckle believes that "most people don't want to do that. They just want to say, 'I'm unhappy.'" Negotiation takes place to set expectations, and that takes time. It involves a discussion of what can be delivered with the available amount of money and whether customers are willing to pay more to get more. If the negotiated service level is met and the customer is still unhappy, new service measures may be needed. Service level agreements draw them into the process. They are required to look at data about what services they are using. Brenckle notes, "It's part of our culture now." Besides customer satisfaction, system reliability and availability are also important.

Service level agreements are not used between IT and UPHS departments. There is only one set of SLAs. Brenckle believes the primary resources are FCG and ACS, so the contract SLAs are sufficient. If UPHS did not outsource IT, he would definitely use SLAs with departments to manage services and expectations.

Vendor Management of Service Level Agreements

Account Manager Weber and his team know the two or three SLAs that are difficult to achieve and focus their efforts on them each month. There are two SLAs that are particularly challenging—network availability and clearing problem tickets.

The SLA for network availability says that no network outages can last more than one hour during the month. The network includes both Philadelphia and areas of New Jersey. Weber believes that major investment by UPHS is needed to prevent outages. The University of Pennsylvania Health System was willing to consider what the business impact of outages was and what measures FCG took to reduce the business impact in determining penalties.

The SLA for resolving problem tickets stipulates that the average for clearing all problem tickets from the help desk for the month cannot exceed ten days. These tickets document problems that do not get resolved on the phone. Two issues have a major impact on clearing tickets. First, UPHS now has more systems, but the staff and budget have stayed the same. First Consulting Group needs to focus on record keeping so that accurate data are available. Second, staff may forget to close a ticket and move on to another problem. If service tickets are not closed when the work is actually done, FCG may not meet an SLA for that month. Weber says, "We have to be on top of every ticket." The project management office (PMO) has primary responsibility for this and for monitoring all SLAs. One PMO staff member works full-time on this task.

Two other SLAs that are achieved on a regular basis, but are difficult, are having project estimates done within five days of the request and meeting project milestones (which cannot be missed without forgiveness from the client).

When Service Level Agreements Are Not Met

Service level agreements set the penalty level when the terms of the SLAs are not met. Penalties are not waived for superior performance on other SLAs at UPHS. Exceeding an SLA for help desk performance does not automatically compensate for not meeting an SLA for network availability. Also, no "bonus" levels or incentive payments are made. Exceeding the SLA metric does not result in a reward. But missing an SLA does not automatically result in a financial penalty, although the contract allows UPHS to impose one and sets a fixed amount. The health system has up to ninety days after receiving the monthly report to ask for a credit to the bill presented by FCG. If Brenckle and Weber disagree on a penalty, the issue can be brought before higher levels of management.

Penalties range from 1/4 percent to 1 percent of the total value of the contract for that month. The University of Pennsylvania Health System can choose to impose a lower penalty, but not a higher one. Brenckle explained the considerations in waiving or collecting a penalty in terms of missing the SLA "a little" and "a lot." Some SLAs are considered very important, so missing one of them even a little is serious and would result in a financial penalty. Missing a less important SLA a little might not result in a penalty. The performance trend is important. The penalty might be waived for one month, but it might be imposed for missing the SLA three months in a row.

The contract allows a penalty to be waived if some event outside of FCG's control happens—for example, a new computer virus appears that the vendors of anti-virus software were not prepared for. However, FCG could be penalized for failing to foresee a situation and taking appropriate measures or if a plan was in place but was not implemented. For example, a power failure may occur that is the fault of the local utility. If FCG did not create all the necessary data backups specified in a recovery plan, however, a penalty could be imposed. The factors Brenckle uses in deciding on a penalty are the impact of the problem on UPHS and whether FCG did all it could to mitigate the effect. A difficult issue is what to do when equipment owned by UPHS fails. Who is to blame? Should FCG have predicted the problem and informed UPHS? What could be done to mitigate the impact?

Brenckle believes SLAs help resolve problems because they get the attention of vendor management. "A little penalty on an SLA has more impact than sitting on a whole bill." Not paying a bill puts it in accounts receivable and is viewed as possibly the fault of the client. A small penalty (1/2 percent or even 1/4 percent) resulting from the failure to meet an SLA results in internal scrutiny that the account manager wants to avoid. "SLAs force visibility inside the company. You don't need massive penalties to get their attention," says Brenckle.

When to Negotiate Service Level Agreements

Brenckle strongly cautions against developing or negotiating SLAs after the vendor contract is signed. "SLAs are easy to negotiate before the contract is signed, but incredibly difficult after the fact. There is no incentive for the vendor. It is not in their interest. They already have the contract. Vendors don't want SLAs. They want flexibility."

Many SLAs have not proved to be important. That said, Brenckle acknowledges, "I've left SLAs in the contract as bargaining chips."

Weber believes that the SLAs are there to protect both the vendor and the client. They establish the minimum level of performance. To the extent that both organizations can learn to work with each other, they become irrelevant.

Data Collection

Some data are collected automatically. For example, an automated system sends consumer satisfaction surveys to staff who use the call center. Mainframes and other computers produce logs concerning their operations. Calls to the help desk are tracked by software called BMC Remedy (www.bmc.com), which records the time of each call, the time to answer, when a service ticket or request is opened, and when it is closed.

Figure CS4-3 shows a monthly report on help desk first-call resolution, indicating the percentage of all calls that result in the problem being resolved during that first call. One such call might be when a user has forgotten a password. Some problems require a visit from a technician (e.g., to replace a monitor) or referral of the user to someone with specialized knowledge about an application. Because these calls could never be resolved on the first call, they are subtracted from the "raw" first calls to determine "contract" first calls (i.e., calls that should be used to determine compliance with SLAs in the contract). Help desk staff mark service tickets for exclusion by indicating why the problem could not be resolved, for example, referral to someone with advanced knowledge of an application. If UPHS staff are concerned that too many service tickets are being excluded, they can review the service tickets and may suggest, for example, further training of call center operators or additions to the technical knowledge base they use.

Figure CS4-4 shows a related metric, help desk average speed to answer within thirty seconds. It is possible that resolving

Figure CS4-3. University of Pennsylvania Health System Help Desk First Call Resolution

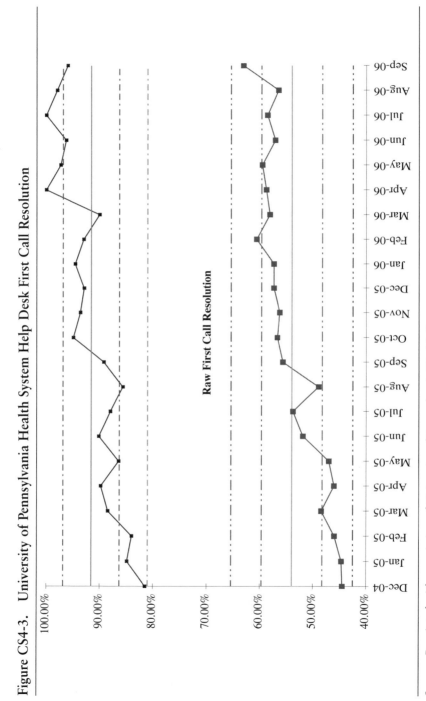

Raw First Call Resolution

Source: Reprinted with permission of University of Pennsylvania Health System.

Figure CS4-4. University of Pennsylvania Health System Help Desk Average Speed to Answer within Thirty Seconds

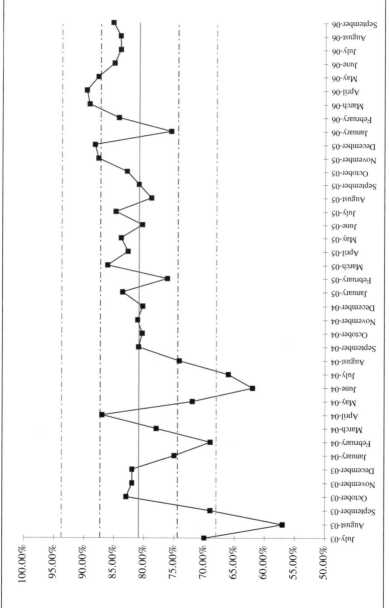

Source: Reprinted with permission of University of Pennsylvania Health System.

more problems on the first call would make fewer operators available at any given time and result in fewer calls answered within thirty seconds. Figures CS4-3 and CS4-4, however, show an upward trend in both metrics. To interpret the numbers, FCG and UPHS staff can look at other metrics, including the total number of calls (table CS4-2). Some of the remaining variability could be due to virus attacks, which cause a sharp increase in the number of calls, affecting both response time and first-call resolution.

A PMO has been established at UPHS, which is now tracking projects using project management software. This is particularly important in the applications development area.

Network availability monitoring is still done manually by looking at calls to the help desk. Some pieces of equipment come with internal monitoring, but not every part of the network is covered.

Reports

A report on all SLAs is now prepared monthly on an Excel spreadsheet and is distributed within IT. First Consulting Group is required to produce this report within five days of the end of the month (a requirement which is itself an SLA). It shows data over a number of months. Review of SLA performance is delegated to a deputy CIO, who meets with FCG staff ten days after the end of the month. Brenckle also expects all of the CIOs of UPHS facilities to be reviewing the SLA data.

Figure CS4-5 shows a report recording the availability of the IDX registration and billing applications for the full-time physician practices from July 2003 to September 2006. Availability would be affected by a network outage or an interface failure. Routine, periodic procedures, including backup and month-end closing, could also take longer than expected, making the application unavailable to users. This is because of the large volume of data. Performance on this SLA would be discussed.

Table CS4-2. University of Pennsylvania Health System Help Desk Service Level Agreements—October 2006

Help Desk Service Levels	Metric	Expected	September 2006	October 2006
First Call Resolution Service Level	Percentage of calls (*within help desk resolution scope*) resolved while user is on initial phone call	65%	95.97%	97.23%
Answer Time Service Level	Percentage of calls answered in less than thirty seconds	80%	85.23%	88.91%
	Total number of help desk calls		9,503	10,067
	Total number of voice mails taken		249	243
	Total number of e-mails taken		2,816	3,350
Repeat Tickets	Percentage resolved the first time solution is implemented	98%	98.61%	98.26%
Call Abandonment Rate	Percentage of calls abandoned	≤5%	1.49%	0.98%
Help Desk Satisfaction Survey	Average score of 4.0 (equal to 80%)	4.0	4.42	4.41

Source: Reprinted with permission of University of Pennsylvania Health System.

Figure CS4-5. University of Pennsylvania Health System IDX Availability

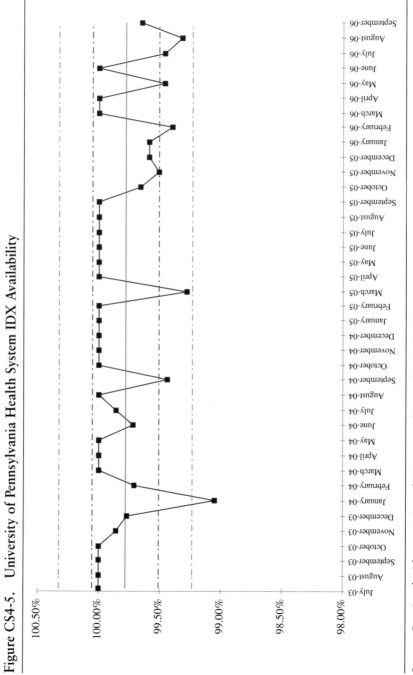

Source: Reprinted with permission of University of Pennsylvania Health System.

A weekly operations meeting (not attended by the CIO) occurs at which issues are discussed, including those reflected in the SLAs, for example, help desk performance. Reports are prepared for this weekly operations meeting. The IT leadership team (e.g., the CIO of one of the facilities) provides summaries when they meet with the leadership of the various entities within UPHS.

The discussion between UPHS and FCG staff at monthly meetings has changed from explaining why FCG missed the SLA to what to do to make sure that the SLA is met in the future.

Cost of Service Level Agreements

Service level agreements cost money, for both FCG and UPHS, but Brenckle feels "management costs money, but if you don't manage well, you're in trouble. Of course you've got to do it. Service level agreements help you manage what you want to deliver. If you have good SLAs, you're going to manage well. Of course it costs money, but the alternative is not delivering." If the collection of the information can be automated, the cost can be driven down a little bit. "It's a small enough cost, so other actions would produce better results, for example, off-shoring some of the work. I'm not looking at how to reduce the cost of SLAs. Service level agreements will help me understand the value of what I'm doing."

Weber estimates that the cost of producing reports and follow-up activity is approximately 1 percent of the contract amount. This does not include the labor costs incurred by UPHS to review and discuss performance.

Future Needs

Brenckle is looking to the new contract to help meet the needs of UPHS as clinical applications grow in importance. "I need more reliability. Five years ago we were running primarily back office systems. Now we are running more clinical systems. My standard for availability now is 99.9 percent of the time. For the new contract, it is 99.999 percent. That's going to cost money. Four hours a month downtime on an order entry system isn't going to be acceptable."

Weber believes that a vendor's strategy should be to provide incredible service. Service level agreements define only the minimum level. They should be in the contract and be simple to monitor. They cannot be used to define and produce exceptional service. That is a question of leadership and management and requires both parties to contribute. The measurement and analysis cannot be done before the contract is signed. "You're not partners until the contract is signed."

Lessons Learned

Brenckle described the following lessons learned over the last five years:

- SLAs are incredibly valuable if you pick the right ones.
- SLAs have to be metrics that you do not have to spend a huge amount of resources to measure.
- SLAs are going to change over time.
- SLAs are a great communications tool. "They can enable and expand the dialogue you need to have about what the expectations are."

Weber described the place of SLAs in this way:

- SLAs are the minimum level of service. In most cases, the SLA is not the level you should be striving to achieve.
- SLAs can become a boat anchor, slowing everything down. They can cause you to throw resources into minimizing the negative. Put in a process to monitor and achieve SLAs, but do not focus on them.
- Manage to achieve excellent client service. Be transparent and candid in discussing how to go beyond the minimum.

References

Herron, David. 2000. *Function points: Their use in software development and maintenance.* Addison-Wesley Professional, November 20. www.awprofessional.com/articles/article.asp?p=19800&rl=1 (accessed December 27, 2006).

University of Pennsylvania Health System. 2001. University of Pennsylvania Health System awards contract for information technology management services. Press release, January 25. www.uphs.upenn.edu/news/News_Releases/jan01/IT_Contract.shtml (accessed December 1, 2006).

Index

(continued)